D0042078

★ ★ ★ ★ ★ ★ ★

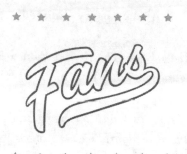

★ ★ ★ ★ ★ ★ ★

Also by Larry Olmsted

Real Food/Fake Food: Why You Don't Know What You're Eating and What You Can Do About It

Getting into Guinness: One Man's Longest, Fastest, Highest Journey Inside the World's Most Famous Record Book

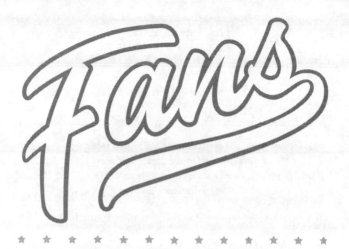

Fans

HOW WATCHING SPORTS
MAKES US HAPPIER, HEALTHIER,
AND MORE UNDERSTANDING

LARRY OLMSTED

ALGONQUIN BOOKS OF CHAPEL HILL   2021

Published by
Algonquin Books of Chapel Hill
Post Office Box 2225
Chapel Hill, North Carolina 27515-2225

a division of
Workman Publishing
225 Varick Street
New York, New York 10014

© 2021 by Larry Olmsted. All rights reserved.
Printed in the United States of America.
Published simultaneously in Canada by Thomas Allen & Son Limited.
Design by Steve Godwin.

Dr. Kristie is based on a real-life MD friend of mine with whom I did
spend a day skiing and broadly discussing these sports topics, including
her actual flirtation with Chicago Bulls fandom, but I have changed her
name, parts of our conversation, and some personal details.

Library of Congress Cataloging-in-Publication Data

Names: Olmsted, Larry, [date]– author.
Title: Fans : how watching sports makes us happier, healthier,
and more understanding / Larry Olmsted.
Description: First edition. | Chapel Hill, North Carolina :
Algonquin Books of Chapel Hill, [2021] |
Includes bibliographical references. | Summary: "Research into
sports fandom makes the sometimes counterintuitive case
for why being a fan is good for us individually and is a force for
positive change in our society"— Provided by publisher.
Identifiers: LCCN 2020041406 | ISBN 9781616208462 (hardcover) |
ISBN 9781643751696 (ebook)
Subjects: LCSH: Sports spectators—Psychology. | Sports—Sociological
aspects. | Sports spectators—Social conditions.
Classification: LCC GV715 .O46 2021 | DDC 306.4/83—dc23
LC record available at https://lccn.loc.gov/2020041406

10 9 8 7 6 5 4 3 2 1
First Edition

For Allison, Zarafa, Chamonix, and sports fans everywhere
—may all your teams do well
(except the Eagles)

CONTENTS

★　★　★　★　★　★　★

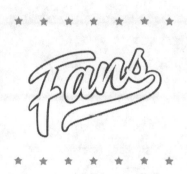

Fans

Pre-Game

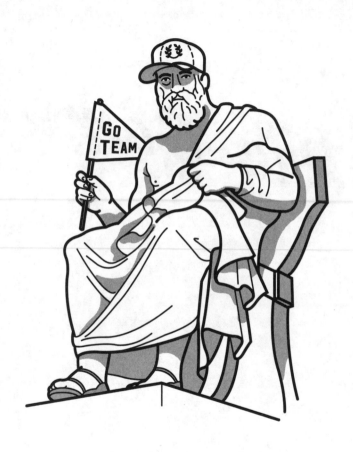

Forty thousand pilgrims would assemble, including
the most distinguished members of Greek society.
Plato and Pythagoras were always in the front seats.
Socrates, Anaxagoras, Demosthenes, Pindar, Herodotus,
and even Diogenes came to the games. The barbarians
could not understand why the Greeks spent so much
time and energy on what seemed to them these childish
pursuits . . . Lucian in one of his dialogues puts the
answer in the mouth of Solon, the famous political
regenerator of Greece and the symbol of wisdom. To this
day Solon's answer is unsurpassed. You would have to be
there, he tells the puzzled barbarian.
—**C.L.R. James on the Olympics in** *Beyond a Boundary*

*S*ince perhaps the beginning of time, or at least of organized athletic games, pundits of all sorts, from many
fields, including science, literature, history, journalism, and

politics, have asked the same question about sports: "why do we care so much?"

Whether or not sports themselves actually matter—a fierce philosophical debate in some quarters—there is no doubt that they are important to us as a society, if only because so many people do care. The forced global absence of organized competition during the 2020 coronavirus pandemic served as a reminder of just how much people love sports and how passionately they miss them when they are gone. We may never know exactly why sports are so important to so many of us, and in this book I decided to ask a different question, one that has received a lot less attention, but one that I consider more enlightening: "what *happens* when we care?"

The world is full of sports fans, and I wanted to know what being a sports fan does to us, individually and collectively.

Let's find out.

Game Time

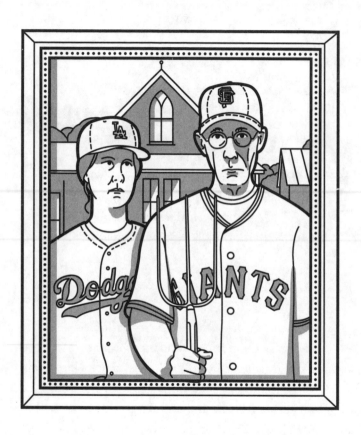

★ ★ ★ ★ ★ ★ ★ ★ ★ ★ ★ ★ ★

Are you a fan? It is altogether to be hoped, for your psychic health and well-being, that you are. In fact, and in spite of the advice and warnings so freely offered by alarmists and loose thinkers, it is equally desirable for your physical health.

—A.A. Brill, MD, "The Why of the Fan"

★ ★ ★ ★ ★ ★ ★ ★ ★ ★ ★ ★ ★

*O*ne of the lengthiest of many conversations I've had in recent years about sports fandom took place just a few weeks before the Super Bowl, the holiest day in American sports. I went skiing in Jackson, Wyoming, home to one of my favorite ski resorts, and also the town where Kristie Hayes, MD, aka Dr. Kristie, practices family medicine—and practices the healthful lifestyle she preaches. In the winter she skis, both at the resort and more often touring in the wilderness backcountry, while in the summer, she hikes and bikes—mountain and road—does yoga, and is a regular at the gym all year round. Before medical school, she did a few years' stint guiding cycling trips for active tour operator Backroads, and during her years at medical school at Dartmouth, part of the college at which I occasionally teach creative writing, we were regular running and road cycling partners. An athletics participant but not a spectator, Dr. Kristie described herself to me, with conviction, as "not a sports fan."

We spent an unusually warm and sunny January day skiing Jackson Hole Mountain Resort, and while riding the chairlifts between runs, she asked what my next book was about. "I'm exploring the effects of sports fandom on individuals and also collectively. I'm looking at what it means to be a sports fan, what it does to us, and what it does to society."

She was simultaneously skeptical and uninterested. But to be polite, she asked, "Why?"

"Sports fans have been dissed. I'd like to set the record straight."

"What do you mean?"

I took a breath. "So many people, here in America and around the globe, identify themselves as being 'sports fans.' In terms of popularity and participation, it's a huge part of our national conversation. The sports section is often the thickest in newspapers, no news broadcast is complete without sports coverage, and sporting events are our most-watched programs of any kind. Yet until very recently, little research has been done into the effects of sports fandom, especially when compared to religion, the most comparable system of widespread group identification and belonging. But the research that has been done, as well as the historical record, overwhelmingly shows that being a sports fan is good for us, good for humanity, and good for the world."

That's a bold claim and one that seemed to surprise Dr. Kristie—and a lot of other people I've talked to.

She thought about it, then shrugged. "I always thought it just seems like a big waste of time."

Here's the thing: when I write the words "sports fans," what picture do you see in your mind? Dr. Kristie likely sees an overweight guy in a team jersey sitting on a couch drinking beer with his overweight jersey-wearing friends, and I'm not surprised. This is how sports fans have been routinely portrayed for decades in the media, on the most popular television sitcoms, in commercials, and in movies.

Scott Simon, NPR *Weekend Edition Saturday* host and former international correspondent, is a devoted, dyed-in-the-wool sports enthusiast who wrote a book called *Home and Away: Memoir of a Fan*. He begins a chapter titled "I'm a Fan" this way: "Fans don't get much respect. In literature and pop culture, advertising and conversation, we are often seen as the anonymously clamorous: bug-eyed and beer-swollen . . ." Longtime ESPN television producer Justine Gubar—and unlikely fan hater, given her profession—described the American sports fan in these words: "That beer-guzzling, jersey-wearing guy headed to his buddy's house to watch football all day. . ."

The corpulent lazy guy is a sitcom staple as well as a commercial fixture (personified by Kevin James's serial sports fan Doug Heffernan, aka *The King of Queens*), but equally unflattering are the most common alternative stereotypes: the loveable jersey-wearing dolt with nothing better to do than watch sports on TV (like Chris Pratt's Andy Dwyer on *Parks and Recreation*) and the screaming, face painted, jersey-wearing maniac (à la NHL Devils fan David Puddy on *Seinfeld*—which also features two other overweight and troubled sports fans in starring roles, George Costanza and Newman). *Saturday Night Live* built a whole franchise of recurring skits around "Da Bears," a group of hard-drinking, hard-eating, jersey-wearing Chicago sports fans. It's set in a bar and portrayed by all the heaviest comedians on the show, plus the occasional overweight guest star. The entertainment industry can't even seem to draw non-obese, non-beer-swilling sports fans—the longest-running sitcom in television history gives us Homer Simpson, and *Family*

Guy stars Peter Griffin, with eighteen seasons behind it. Both shows are animated, hilarious, and still on the air.

The movies haven't been especially kind to sports fans, either, though for the most part Hollywood has simply ignored them. No amount of permutations of the words "sports, spectators, fans, and movies" could google me up any kind of list, compilation, or discussion of movies focused on sports fans, because there are, as far as I can tell, only four of note—versus literally thousands on sports in general (Wikipedia lists five just for the subcategory of "Greyhound Racing"). This mostly undistinguished quartet includes *Big Fan*, a comedic look at the rather bleak life of a football-obsessed (and, of course, beefy and jersey-wearing) parking garage attendant whose every waking moment revolves around the New York Giants and sports talk radio. In this case, the *Big Fan* of the title is a double entendre referring to both the depth of his passion and his physique.

It gets worse. *Green Street* features Elijah Wood as an improbable Harvard journalism student who decides to move to London and join a gang of soccer hooligans who live for violent brawling with rival fans. If you are going to produce one movie about fans every decade or so, why wouldn't you opt for this particularly unlikely plot, right? But we have yet to hit rock bottom. The best-known example and cream of this way-off-base crop is *The Fan*, with

Robert De Niro as an insane, down-on-his-luck, knife sales-man (?!) and baseball junkie who stalks the star player of the San Francisco Giants, played by Wesley Snipes. In the process, he becomes increasingly unhinged, slashing, beat-ing, stabbing, kidnapping, and killing his way through the movie (and, yes, he dons a jersey).

By far the most palatable of the bunch is *Fever Pitch*, a romantic comedy remake of an English movie adapted from the excellent Nick Hornby soccer memoir of the same name. The depiction of fandom in the entertain-ment world is an ever-evolving continuum, and *Fever Pitch* occupies higher ground. Its stars, Jimmy Fallon and Drew Barrymore, eventually overcome the romantic gulf caused by Fallon's obsessive baseball fandom, and in a Hollywood twist, Fallon is portrayed as neither down on his luck, insane, nor obese (though he frequently dons jerseys).

★ ★ ★ ★ ★ ★ ★ ★ ★ ★ ★ ★ ★ ★

**Are sports fans lazy? One of the most common criticisms
of sports fans involves the perception that they
are lazy . . . The criticism that sports fans are lazy
has not held up well to empirical investigation.
—*Sports Fans: The Psychology and
Social Impact of Spectators***

★ ★ ★ ★ ★ ★ ★ ★ ★ ★ ★ ★ ★ ★

All of this creates a stereotype that feeds Dr. Kristie's image of sports fandom as time wasted. I decided at that moment, there on the ski slope, that I was going to try to change her mind—which meant she was about to spend the rest of the day talking about sports, whether she wanted to or not. Or maybe the rest of the weekend.

SPORTS FANS ARE HAPPIER PEOPLE

"You have a day off today. Why did you come skiing?" I ask Dr. Kristie as we are getting off the chairlift.

"Because it makes me happy."

"Is that important? I mean from a medical perspective?" This launches the good doctor into a consideration of mental health, and "of course" is her inevitable conclusion. She even quotes some of the countless studies and decades of research that have proven the mental and physical health benefits of happiness and tells me that this is being viewed as more essential than ever in an era of greatly increased awareness of depression, loneliness, and other emotional maladies.

In his fascinating book, *Blue Mind,* Wallace J. Nichols, PhD, a researcher at the California Academy of Sciences, quotes the Dalai Lama—"The purpose of our lives is to be happy"—and concludes that "with all the benefits of happiness, who would disagree?" He writes, " . . . greater

individual happiness has been shown to make our relationships better; help us be more creative, productive, and
effective at work (thereby bringing us higher incomes); give
us greater self-control and ability to cope; make us more
charitable, cooperative, and empathetic; boost our immune,
endocrine, and cardiovascular systems; lower cortisol and
heart rate; decrease inflammation, slow disease progres-
sion and increase longevity . . . Happy people demonstrate
better cognition and attention, make better decisions, take
better care of themselves, and are better friends, colleagues,
neighbors, spouses, parents, and citizens."

★ ★ ★ ★ ★ ★ ★ ★ ★ ★ ★

**People's lives are enriched—there's very clear research
showing that the more you identify with a local
sports team, the better your social psychological
health is. This stuff matters to people.
—Daniel L. Wann, PhD, "The ABCs of Sports Fandom,"
Murray State University**

★ ★ ★ ★ ★ ★ ★ ★ ★ ★ ★

No one has studied the psychological ramifications of
sports fandom more than Dr. Daniel L. Wann, a psychology professor at Murray State University in Kentucky. The

modern pioneer in the field, Wann has authored or co-authored close to two hundred significant journal articles and book chapters, several books, and more than one hundred papers presented at conferences globally. His first academic paper specifically on sports spectators was published in 1989, and he jokes that when he began studying sports fans as a doctoral candidate at the University of Kansas, so little had been done in this field that not only did he not have a road map for research, but that "there was no road." Wann had to create a new kind of questionnaire to identify fans and measure their level of fandom for his studies, and his Sports Spectator Identification Scale, or SSIS (now revised and expanded), is today the gold standard for researchers worldwide. "I can remember thinking, not only is there not a scale to improve upon, there's not anyone writing about this to give us ideas for what the scale should be in the first place."

In his three-plus decades of research, he's undertaken countless studies of men and women, young and old, fans of very different professional and amateur sports all around the world. The bottom line? For those who "identify with a sports team," as he defines a fan, he has found no less than twenty-four specific mental health benefits. Some of the biggest pluses that Wann and now other researchers have found include higher self-esteem; fewer bouts of depression; less alienation; lower levels of loneliness; higher levels of extroversion; higher levels of satisfaction with their social lives; more friends; higher levels of trust in others; more vigor and less fatigue; less anger; less confusion; less tension; greater frequency of experiencing positive emotions; and more conscientiousness. These sound very similar to Dr. Nichols's general happiness markers.

In 2019 Wann presented a university psychology colloquium called "The ABCs of Sport Fandom: What We Know and Where We Should Go" and explained it this way:

> What we call the ABCs of psychology are affect, behavior, and cognition, or how we feel, what we do, and how we think. Sport fandom—the fact that we follow teams and sports and players—really does impact our emotional state. It really does impact what we do, what we think, how we perceive the world. The big picture is that one thing fandom does is it helps to meet basic psychological needs, things like the need to belong, to feel a sense of connection to those around us. If you're in Murray, Kentucky, and you're a Racers basketball fan, it's hard to feel lonely. It's hard to feel alienated.
>
> But it can also provide a sense of distinctiveness that can allow people to feel unique. Our ultimate

goal in life is to fit in, while standing out. We want to fit in, but we don't want to be exactly like everyone else. So, you can be a sports fan that follows the local team and fits in, but you can also be a fan of a team [or sport] that maybe not a whole lot of people in that part of the country follow, so you can fit in but be different, unique, and distinct as well. People can use sports to meet these very powerful psychological needs.

★ ★ ★ ★ ★ ★ ★ ★ ★ ★ ★ ★ ★ ★

Sports are very emotional, and they do bring people together. You can be watching a game on TV and still feel affinity for the people in the stands and solidarity with them, and you get the sense that you're one of a group of people, a community. Even if you're sitting in front of a TV by yourself somewhere, you still feel as if you are participating.
—Dartmouth Visiting Professor Peter DeShazo, as told to the author

★ ★ ★ ★ ★ ★ ★ ★ ★ ★ ★ ★ ★ ★

A feeling of belonging leads to other mental health benefits, as the *New York Times* put it, "Sports fans suffer fewer bouts of depression and alienation than do people who are uninterested in sports."

Most of sports' psychological pluses accrue in two inter-related areas: belonging and self-esteem. The advantages of being part of a community of sports fans supporting a particular team are very real, as Dr. Wann described, "The benefits of social support are not limited to one's psychology but, rather, also predict both physical health and longevity of life."

Most researchers define a sports fan as someone who supports and follows at least one team in one sport or league, what Dr. Wann refers to as "identifying with a team." But it is possible to be a sports fan without having any favorite team—those spectators whose sportive interest is devoted entirely to individual competitions, such as tennis, boxing, or golf, though this is a small subset. In this book I'll largely stick with the more commonly researched team-based parameters, but with a few caveats. First, when data comes from the fans' perspective, such as polls asking whether they consider themselves fans, the definition really does not matter because the opinion is one of self-evaluation. If you say you're a sports fan, that's good enough for me. Secondly, as we'll see, the majority of sports fans support more than one team, so Wann's definition is a minimum, not the norm. Finally, while the psychologist's definition would exclude fans of non-team sports from their data, I think it will be clear that many of the benefits we'll be looking at would—especially physical health benefits—still accrue to followers of skiing, track and field, and so on.

I use the term "sports fandom" a lot, and it is different from spectator sports, as fans are a much bigger part of the total equation than athletes. Without fandom, sports has no platform. Nearly eighty million living, breathing fans attended Major League Baseball games in person in 2017, but in sharp contrast, there were just 877 players on rosters (including those injured, disabled, or suspended). When newly elected President Nelson Mandela enlisted the national rugby team to alleviate racial tensions, prevent the looming possibility of a bloody civil war, and unite Blacks and Whites in post-apartheid South Africa, the sport was a tool to reach the hearts and minds of much of the country's population: rugby fans. No matter how devoted they were to Mandela's cause, the twenty-three professional athletes could hardly have made a difference on their own—it was the millions of fans who chose peaceful reconciliation. The Super Bowl–winning quarterback would never get to hoist the trophy and exclaim "I'm going to Disney World!" if people did not want to pay to go to games and watch football. But they do want to, which is ultimately good news for all of us.

A joint global project between a researcher at Temple University and peers in the UK and Australia analyzed 135 academic and research papers on sport spectators published around the world between 1990 and 2014 and concluded that, "Sport spectating provides numerous benefits." They grouped these into five distinct mental health well-being categories: positive emotions, engagement, relationships, meaning, and accomplishment.

"Humans are inherently tribal creatures, and this is a way to have a tribe," wrote economics professor Kevin Quinn, author of *Sports and Their Fans*. So many of the psychological advantages sports fans enjoy come from this sense of belonging to a community, that today sports fandom plays an even more vital role in our happiness than ever before. That is because other long-standing social gathering networks, from fraternal organizations to bowling leagues, have slipped away, and organized religious participation is waning. In contrast to these other large-scale social activities, though, our love of sports shows no sign of slowing down. The Super Bowl remains unfailingly the single most-watched show of the year, regardless of what else occurs, and several other major sporting events typically round out the top ten. In 2018, these included *Sunday Night Football*, whose average Nielsen ratings put it third on the list, and *Thursday Night Football* at number ten.

> For tens of millions of Americans, sport was not leisure anymore . . . Sport had become a national obsession, a new cultural currency, a kind of social cement binding a diverse society together. Instead of work, family, or religion, increasingly large numbers of Americans were choosing sport as the focus of their lives.
> —**Randy Roberts and James Olson, *Winning is the Only Thing: Sports in America Since 1945***

More than a decade ago, Dr. Wann wrote, "The finding that team identification [fandom] has direct positive effects on psychological well-being is particularly important in light of the fact that many traditional connections to society appear to be declining. Affiliations with others stemming from religious institutions, work-related organizations, and relationships with extended family members have all have shown reduced numbers in recent years. It has been argued that identification with sports teams may serve to replace the traditional but declining social ties as members of society attempt to reestablish and maintain their social connectedness. Consequently, these identifications become more vital to the maintenance of psychological well-being." Sports fills a void.

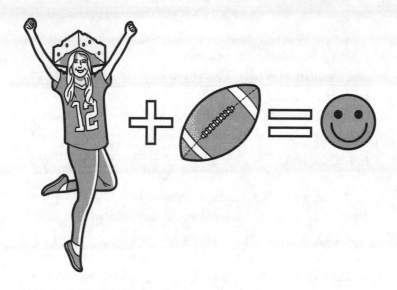

Dr. Wann told me this has only been amplified by tele-commuting and remote offices, reducing the need for a shared workspace, where people engaged in much of their social interaction. What had become the last widespread, communal, daily gathering place in our society is now threatened, and this technological isolation flies in the face of human nature, which still needs community. That is one reason many people who work from home gravitate to group tables in hotel lobbies and coffee shops, so they can work alone in the "company" of strangers.

I had read much of Dr. Wann's work, but instead of answers, some of the studies just begat more questions. So I traveled to Kentucky to attend the annual university sports psychology conference he co-hosts for researchers and graduate students. I arranged to meet him in person for lunch the first day and not knowing how much one-on-one time we would have, I jumped right in with the bottom line: "You've been studying this for over thirty years. How important is sports fandom to our health, and how sure are you of it?"

"I can remember the first time we ever found this fan effect—we were prepping for another study that was unrelated, but in this correlation study I saw the link between fandom and these positive benefits like higher self-esteem and less alienation and I was really surprised. I had thought that being a fan was just being a fan, a sometimes expensive and sometimes disappointing hobby. But I started looking into it and since then there have been many more studies, with teens and adults, all over the world, with the same results. I am now 150 percent convinced of the benefits of sports fandom."

Researchers Chaeyoon Lim of the University of Wisconsin–Madison and Robert Putnam of Harvard University studied this community-induced happiness effect among active members of religious groups, calling the resulting benefit "social capital." Reaching beyond this, the psychological benefits of fandom are potentially life-saving. Karolina Krysinska and Karl Andriessen have been studying suicide prevention for a quarter of a century, and concluded that being a fan and following a team, "creates camaraderie, a sense of belongingness and being cared for and can result in sports-related 'pulling together' which might protect against suicide." Wann and his colleagues looked into the duo's suicide prevention claims and found that other impartial empirical research substantiated it. "Given that sports fandom is directly related to lower levels of alienation and loneliness, it feeds right into this," he told me. "Feeling more connected and less alienated are known correlators toward being less suicidal."

★ ★ ★ ★ ★ ★ ★ ★ ★ ★ ★ ★ ★

**If you are lonely and depressed . . .
find a sports team to support!
—Association for Applied Sport Psychology
press release**

★ ★ ★ ★ ★ ★ ★ ★ ★ ★ ★ ★ ★

SPORTS AS ENTERTAINMENT

"Okay, I get how watching sports makes fans happy," said Dr. Kristie. "But when I get a break from work and my child goes to sleep and I need some 'me time,' I binge episodes of my favorite series." She tore through addictive dramas like *Breaking Bad* and *The Americans* and now challenged me: "Isn't that the same thing? Why wouldn't I get the same benefits?"

Even though the mental health benefits of sports fandom have been proven, you might wonder, like Dr. Kristie, if all forms of entertainment could offer the same results. For example, what if reading makes you happy? Or going to the movies? Or being a fan of *Game of Thrones*?

But sports are different from most other kinds of entertainment for a variety of reasons. While viewing spectator sports actually encourages physical activity and fitness (more on this soon), avid consumption of shows via Netflix, Hulu, and the like seem to discourage it. While sports fans reap big wins from being part of a community—even when viewing alone—binge-watching can isolate and alienate us and replace socialization time. A 2017 study by researchers at Michigan State University found a link between binge-watching and "poor lifestyle behaviors such as opting for unhealthy meals, unhealthy snacks, and sedentary behaviors." In a *Washington Post* feature on the current research into this, health journalist Jenna Birch notes that, "According to several experts, binge-watching can affect your cardiovascular system, your vision, your socialization, and your sleep patterns—all of which can lead to other problems." These range from increased risk of heart disease, stroke, type 2 diabetes, and deep-vein thrombosis to neck and shoulder pain, headaches, and blurred vision to social isolation that adversely affects relationships.

But even if you do not binge-watch, sports viewing may be different from other diversions. "Sports fans are not just simply sitting around and watching a game, sort of mindlessly being entertained. It's not like they're watching their favorite sitcom or reality TV show," said Wann. "It really impacts the human experience a lot more than I think a lot of people understand."

Sports are by their nature completely unpredictable and always new. While there may be twists and turns and even shocks in their dramatic journeys, in most cases we recognize that James Bond or the *Mission Impossible* team is going to save the world before we walk into the theater—we know which team is going to win.

———★★★★★★★★★★★———

I believe and hope to prove that cricket and football were the greatest cultural influences in nineteenth-century Britain, leaving far behind Tennyson's poems, Beardsley's drawings, and concerts of the Philharmonic Society.
—Historian, Professor, and *Beyond a Boundary* author C.L.R. James

———★★★★★★★★★★★———

"[T]here is one crucial dimension in which sports differ markedly in their structure and texture from language, the arts, theater, music, and many other creative categories that so enrich human life: its unscriptedness. Indeed, this is absolutely essential to all modern sports . . . The uncertainty of results is arguably *the* greatest difference between sports and related human activities that are very similar to sports, notably entertainment . . . No matter how much one contestant—team or individual—is superior to the other, winning the contest is never a forgone conclusion," writes Professor Andrei Markovits and his co-author Lars Rensmann in their book *Gaming the World*. Dr. Markovits, an Arthur F. Thurnau Professor at the University of Michigan, has researched "sports cultures" for over thirty years, and by this he is referring to the social framework wherein people "follow" sports, rather than participate in them.

The reason advertisers love sports above other programming—now more than ever—is because they are the last major form of broadcast or digitally delivered entertainment most people still watch live and in real time. Accidentally hearing the final score or result ruins part of the unscripted nature of the experience. No one waits seventeen weeks to binge-watch the previous NFL season. (Though classic sports did finally get a binge-watching "moment in the sun" during the 2020 coronavirus pandemic, when networks and cable stations re-aired old—sometimes very old—games, especially former NCAA March Madness competitions, reflecting the month in which most live sports were suspended.)

"The bewildering complexity of today's best TV content repels casual consumption and therefore common conversation," argued Michael Serazio from the stage at the 2019 Sport at the Service of Humanity Conference, co-sponsored by the Vatican Pontifical Council for Culture. Dr. Serazio is a professor at Boston University and the author of *The Power of Sports: Media and Spectacle in American Culture*. "You can't simply drop in on the *Game of Thrones* season finale without

massive time investment beforehand. But Game Seven
of the NBA finals is considerably less befuddling, even if
you didn't catch the previous six. In short, peak TV [the
recently popular term for the current digitally-driven iter-
ation of the 'Golden Age' of television] is great for art but
less so for widespread social communion. Sports, on the
other hand, still offer the glue of collective conscience that
the acid of modern life has otherwise dissolved. Sports tells
us what time it is, and anchors players and fans alike in the
present moment, concentrating vast shared psychic energy
on events unfolding right now."

Something else that makes sports spectating distinct
from many other forms of entertainment is its sense of
community and the belonging it creates while we are consuming it. Even though science fiction or fantasy fans can
be just as passionate about their interest as sports fans, and
might get dressed up in costume and go to ComicCon or
wait in line all night to see the latest release, the nature
of the way we watch sports differentiates it. When I asked
Dr. Wann whether being a devoted Harry Potter fan would
produce the same benefits and sense of belonging to something bigger, he told me, "The difference is that you experience sports fandom collectively, but while you can go to
a book club and talk about a book after the fact, you read
it alone. You can be a *Star Wars* fan and talk to other fans
about it, but not during the movie." In fact, if you watched

a movie the way most of us watch sports, you would quickly get thrown out of the theater. Sports is dramatically singular in this respect—it would be odd for people watching together *not* to constantly analyze and discuss the action in real time.

Furthermore, when you watch *Breaking Bad* at home, or on your phone, you are not bombarded with images of tens of thousands of people just like you, many in hats and T-shirts adorned with "your" team logo, watching in the stands, enjoying the action and cheering along, exactly as you are doing at the same time. In spectator sports the audience is part of the show, frequently onscreen, and this serves as a constant reinforcement of the sense of community sports fans enjoy so much. While there a few exceptions, such as attending a rock concert, most other popular entertainment simply does not have this kind of audience participation.

Both the overall happiness benefits of sports and the connection to the stadium audience through the TV screen were lost for the longest period in modern history during the 2020 coronavirus pandemic. To one of the world's leading researchers of fan psychology, Dr. Rick Grieve, director of Western Kentucky University's Doctor of Psychology in Applied Psychology program, the two are importantly interrelated: "Spectator sports are one of the top two (the other being religion) areas in which Americans socialize with others," even if we do not know them or only see them through a camera lens. "We make connections with people who we see wearing merchandise with the insignia of our favorite team, even if those are only momentary connections. We can all come together as a community—regardless of race, ethnicity, gender, sexual identification, or any other sort of divisor—and be a fan of the team."

That connection between fans at the game and those at home had long received little attention outside of sports psychology circles, but it suddenly became a hot topic of conversation as major spectator sports returned without in-person spectators. Music and pop culture specialist Jody Rosen, a contributing writer to the *New York Times'* Sunday magazine, followed the fast return of Germany's high-profile and top-tier Bundesliga pro soccer league, and penned "The Eerie Sound of Sports Without Fans." He concluded that "Fans watching at home need the fans in the stands; without them, a crucial life force drains from the games. The roar of the crowd is not mere background noise. It's the music of sports—the soundtrack that transforms a ballgame into a melodrama, must-see TV, the greatest show on earth."

But even if fans miss the extra boost that having anonymous members of their community on the screen in front of them brings, it may turn out to be just a minor bump in the road of sports fandom. "Sports provides people an outlet for their fears, worries, and stressors. I do think that a return to sports—even without fans in the seats—will provide an escape from the hassles surrounding working from home, alternative teaching, and reduced hours (or no hours) at work," Dr. Grieve told me. Molly Roberts, an editorial writer for the *Washington Post*, put the return of baseball and basketball during the coronavirus pandemic this way: "The show must go on, apparently, because we don't know what we'd do without it. We're looking to sports for a grand reprise of our regular lives in a very irregular summer."

The cessation and return of live sports during the pandemic clearly showed how vitally important they remain in our lives, and how starved fans were for them. As Germany's Bundesliga soccer league returned to the pitch for the first time after the pandemic pause, the *New York Times* reported that, "In Germany, the 37.7 market share for the time period easily eclipsed the Bundesliga's previous record," and predicted that as ratings were finalized, it was "almost certain to end up as the most-watched German match ever." Here in the US, where the league airs on the Fox Sports FS1 channel, viewership was 564 percent higher than the last Bundesliga game the cable channel showed before the shutdown, and nearly six times the league's US average.

When our "national game," baseball, returned in July, the results were even more demonstrative. The season opener drew a record 4.4 million viewers, up from 1.2 million the year before. It was ESPN's largest opening night audience, and the most-watched regular season MLB game on any network in a decade. Fans did not stop there—the second game, a West Coast matchup that did not begin until after 10 p.m. Eastern time, became ESPN's most-watched regular season late night game ever, averaging 2.7 million viewers.

While opinions on the effects of the interruption vary, virtually every expert I spoke with about sports and the pandemic agreed with the basic premise that being a sports fan can help make us happier.

I asked Dr. Wann which of the twenty-four mental health benefits of sports fandom he had identified was most important to us as society. "There are other biggies, but if you pressed me to pick just one face of fandom that belongs on the Mt. Rushmore of psychology, it's the sense of belonging. It's been proven to be very positive and it ties into a lot of other good things." He believes this group identification extends beyond the game-viewing experience and into everyday life, such as seeing fellow fans at the supermarket the next day. Maybe the same would be true when *Lord of the Rings* or Green Day fans encountered one another, but the reality is that the prevalence of sports team apparel over concert tees or *Walking Dead* logo baseball hats makes the shared sports fan experience much more common.

★ ★ ★ ★ ★ ★ ★ ★ ★ ★ ★ ★

We call it the "head nod," when you're walking someplace
and you see someone else in your team's hat and you
just look at each other and nod, and what you're
saying is "you and I are connected, it doesn't matter
who you are or where you're from."
**—Former NFL, MLB, and Current NHL Executive
Brian Killingsworth, as told to the author**

★ ★ ★ ★ ★ ★ ★ ★ ★ ★ ★ ★

"Of course it makes you happier," Dr. Leeja Carter told
me when I asked whether the touted mental health benefits of fandom held up to scrutiny. Because it sounded
almost too good to be true, I still had my doubts. Dr. Carter
is a Fulbright scholar, an assistant professor at Long Island
University–Brooklyn, and head of the Diversity & Inclusion
Council for the Association for Applied Sport Psychology,
a thirty-three-year-old global organization of sports psychologists in 298 countries. "When it comes to being a
fan, and what does that do you for, I think there are many
benefits. It gives you another community, a community of
like-minded people who are engaged in something. It gives
people a shared experience, something to look forward to,
and within that community, to talk about something that
is very impassioned. Just from my own family experience,

we are huge Phillies and Eagles fans. My sisters wear Eagles jerseys every single day, and I'm not exaggerating. I guarantee you one of them has on an Eagles shirt right now. That makes them feel like they are part of a larger community, which is similar to the feeling of religion."

In 1958, the New York Giants played the Baltimore Colts in Yankee Stadium, in what most sports historians believe is the defining moment of football's ascendancy to its current supremacy among American sports. Marking the arrival of the sport in prime time, using the newly popular technology of live television, it became the most-watched football game thus far in history, with some 45 million tuning in. Most importantly, many were watching a professional football game for the first time, and it turned out to be an epic, action-packed, nail-biter for the ages, which in turn birthed many of the conventions of modern sports television.

Mark Bowden, the author of *Blackhawk Down* and other bestsellers, wrote a book about this match-up aptly titled *The Best Game Ever*. He compared the way we now watch sports not with movies or music or other forms of popular entertainment, but rather with the most significant achievements, tragedies, and historic events of our lifetime, and I think he is on to something: "There was a sense throughout Yankee Stadium and in homes all over America that something truly memorable was unfolding . . . The nation was experiencing what was still a new kind of human experience, a truly communal live national event, something made possible by the new medium. In future years the phenomenon would become familiar, but no less powerful, as the nation gathered to watch rocket launches, the aftermath of assassinations, a magnificent civil rights speech, an astronaut stepping onto the moon, a presidential resignation, and someday even the slow-speed highway chase in Los Angeles of a former NFL star charged with a double murder . . ."

More than half a century later, at the Sport at the Service of Humanity Conference, Professor Serazio explained how this trend has continued, "Last year sports made up eighty-nine of the top one hundred most-watched TV programs . . . being in the moment is incredibly valuable for advertisers in the time-shifting age of DVRs and streaming, but it is also existentially critical for the rest of us. Unlike most all forms of entertainment and pop culture, sports resist being 'on demand.' It instead demands of you co-presence with others at specifically scheduled intersections. There's something sacred in that communal immediacy, that ephemeral ecstasy of everyone seeming to be on the same page as the scroll of history unfolds. The most people in the history of humankind to share the same experience at the same time are audiences for recent international sporting events."

SPORTS AND OUR BRAINS: PART 1

*B*ack on the mountain, Dr. Kristie and I stopped for a mid-morning hot chocolate break, ducking out of winter for a few minutes. I could see her mind churning as she processed all the ways that fandom makes us happier. "I hadn't thought of sports and our brains that way. But it makes sense," she admitted.

Sensing a chink in her armor, I was determined to win over my friend, so I took this opportunity to pile on. First I told her about the studies showing that sports fans maintain better cognitive processing as their gray matter ages. Dr. Alan Castel, a psychology professor at UCLA, where he runs the memory and lifespan cognition lab, wrote, "[T]he best thing we can do to maintain brain fitness is to exercise," and explained how watching baseball does just that. It is what Castel calls a "cognitively-demanding" activity: "following sports involves a lot of mental processing and cognitive operations. We draw on prior knowledge, the rules of the game (semantic memory), and need to constantly update information (the score, who is injured, what player is on a hot streak). Perhaps more importantly, baseball is a game, with uncertain outcomes. Our brains often get excited when it comes to playing games, and especially so if you have personal connections to the teams or outcome . . . From a personal perspective, I have often spent a great deal of time talking to many older and wiser adults about sports. My eighty-four-year-old father-in-law recites lineups from the game last night, as well as from the 1954 Cubs."

Fans will excitedly discuss and dissect virtually any aspect of sports, but an especially popular and passionate rabbit hole many love to go down is "Monday morning quarter-backing." While certainly not limited to NFL football, and maybe even more common in the college game, which would make it "Sunday morning quarterbacking." Anyone who has ever tuned into sports talk radio knows that fans eagerly embrace the concept of second-guessing, often examining the minutiae of coaches' decisions and players' actions in painstaking detail.

While some of this is just bitterness over outcomes or anger directed to less favored coaches or players, many of these fans really know their stuff and informed post-game analysis requires firing up their brain cells to do some highly critical thinking. After all, truly understanding the Cover 2 defense or arcane baseball statistics popularized in the book and movie *Moneyball* is an impressive intellectual, or at least cerebral, exercise. My personal knowledge of baseball numbers is frozen in time in the early eighties, and as such, is limited to stats like earned run average (ERA) and batting average (BA). For the fans who grasp modern sabermetrics and can throw around concepts like weighted on base average (wOBA), weighted runs created plus (wRC+), on-base plus slugging plus (OPS+), fielding independent pitching (FIP), and batting average on balls in play (BABIP) in angry post-game calls to sports radio hosts, more power to them.

A 2008 study by University of Chicago researchers also found that turning the TV to a game is a workout for your brain: "[W]atching sports might improve your communication and help you stay organized." Sian Beilock, an associate psychology professor at the University of Chicago, studied three groups: hockey players, hockey fans, and people who had never seen or played the sport. She recorded their brain function while watching hockey, and found that watching sports was a lot closer to actually playing than previously thought—the region of the brain associated with planning and controlling actions is activated when players and fans listen to conversations about their sport, in a way that is lost upon non-fans. "What I think our research suggests is a strong connection between the mind and the body. When

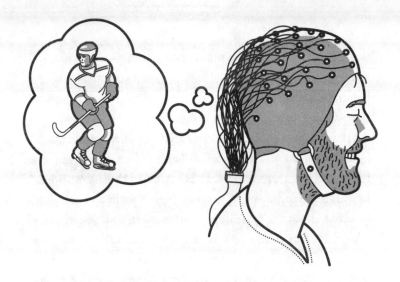

we are sitting on the couch watching a football game or a hockey game, our brain is actually playing the game itself in a way." Better language skills were among the other demonstrated benefits.

Journalist Lizette Borreli pursued this same line of reasoning for *Medical Daily*: "The spectating brain is also a playing brain when it comes to sports. When we're watching sports, it feels as if we're actually playing in the game. We begin to place ourselves in the 'athlete's shoes' thanks to mirror neurons primarily found in the right side of the brain. These cells allow us to reflect and connect to someone else's movements without verbal communication . . . Previous studies have found that when we see a familiar action, our mirror neurons activate and fire for exactly as long as the observed action. This is what allows us to instantly understand the action, its goal, and even the emotions linked to it."

It turns out that doing controlled studies with fans of multiple teams is much more difficult than fans of just one team, so for years researchers have selected those who "identify highly" with a single team as their baseline sports fan. But that is not the typical fan, and more than a dozen years ago Dr. Wann first noted in one of his studies that, "the impact of multiple ties to local sports teams is unknown. If high levels of identification with one local sports team are associated with psychological well-being, would identifying strongly with multiple teams lead to an even better state of mental health?" This is an important question, because when Western Kentucky's Dr. Grieve studied how many teams the average college sports fan followed, using a mixed-gender population, the answer was not one but rather around six: three very closely, two moderately, and one and a half a little bit. Certainly, most people I know follow more than one team in more than one sport.

Dr. Wann recently completed his first study focused on the more typical fan, those of multiple teams, but he started with just two, not six. He explained that each team you add to the equation (are you a fan of two teams or three or four or five?) makes the number of subjects required exponentially higher to the point where testing for fans of six teams becomes prohibitively difficult. Still, the results were impressive. As he told me, "We assessed identification with two teams, and put subjects into four groups based on their level of fandom for one, the other, or both. The group that identified highly with both teams had crazy high mental health scores—several standard deviations above what you would expect randomly in the population," and even higher than fans of single teams. Because that is still based on substantially fewer team identifications than most spectators have in the real world, it's reasonable to surmise that these benefits, "crazy high mental health scores," might well be even greater for most sports fans.

Dr. Wann reminded me that fandom studies have generally been done based on team sports, which are the most popular sports in this country, at the high school, college, and professional levels, and worldwide (in the United States, football, basketball, and baseball are the top three, everywhere else it is soccer, soccer, and soccer, along with extremely popular cricket). But he believes the findings would be similar for individual sports such as golf, tennis, or swimming. He also noted that in real life many, if not most, sports fans follow a mix—plenty of football fans also watch golf, for example.

★ ★ ★ ★ ★ ★ ★ ★ ★ ★ ★ ★

Despite the fact that sports fans are everywhere . . . studies that have been done are piecemeal . . . but even so, they show that many of the basic assumptions about fans are wrong . . . there's even evidence to suggest that fans may actually be smarter on average than nonfans.
—Warren St. John, *Rammer Jammer Yellow Hammer*

★ ★ ★ ★ ★ ★ ★ ★ ★ ★ ★ ★

"What else have you got?" Dr. Kristie asked. I hoped I was winning her over. At least I wasn't losing her.

Well, college students who are sports fans also have higher GPAs, better graduation rates, and higher incomes upon graduating. Many fans I spoke with believed that their love of sports helped further their professional careers and bring them success. One sports-mad casino executive I spoke to in Las Vegas applies lessons learned from watching team sports to his own office group and told me, "Sports has definitely had a positive impact on my life. Sports has definitely made me better at my job."

Elle Kaplan is the founder and CEO of New York-based LexION Capital, a fiduciary wealth management firm—and, not incidentally, did her undergraduate study at the University of Michigan, whose Wolverines play in the nation's largest sports stadium, "The Big House." Kaplan uses sports lessons as metaphors for business success and wrote about several such fan-relatable strategies in an article for CNBC. Most notably, she held up the example of baseball's record-holding ironman, Cal Ripkin, who wowed fans nonstop through three decades, and boasts the longest consecutive-games-played streak in history, at 2,632. "Consistency carries over into several aspects of the business world," Kaplan noted. "It begins with your work ethic . . . When asked what mentality fueled his consistency, [Ripkin] replied, 'Any day could have been my greatest day playing the game.' . . . When you are at work, remember that what you put into each business today has the potential to yield incredible results down the road."

SPORTS AND OUR BRAINS: PART 2

*A*s I talked to various researchers about their studies, I started to wonder just how are they actually conducted? How exactly do they collect all this data?

When Professor Serazio wanted to learn about fan attitudes toward the mingling of sports and politics, he utilized traditional polling techniques and conducted a national telephone study, using statistical parameters to ensure a random sample representative of the general population. Most psychologists use written questionnaires, a faster and cheaper way to get data than doing actual interviews. Sometimes these are on college or high school campuses, sometimes at sporting events, sometimes more widespread, either through the mail or via multiple data collection points.

"We've done it lots of ways," said Dr. Wann, who has likely conducted more fan studies than anyone. "Ideally it's a combination of here in the lab and in the field at sporting events. I like gathering data at sporting events but, man, it's hard."

For events, he typically employs graduate student researchers and has them work the stands pre-game, handing out fliers stating something like, "We're doing a study, if you are willing to participate, please come to this place in the stadium after the game." Then students with clipboards distribute and collect written surveys. Dr. Wann has even employed his wife as volunteer labor. Sometimes he hits the season ticket lounges where, depending on the venue, there is often a captive audience. "In college, I love men's and women's doubleheaders, because there is usually a twenty-minute break where people have nothing to do, and they are happy to take a survey."

Some researchers do meta-studies, culling through numerous studies that have been done by other researchers around the world and aggregating results. And there are definitely some more invasive approaches. Australian doctors inserted fine needles into subjects' nerves to precisely monitor metabolic responses while watching sporting scenes. Lots of researchers have used MRIs or other brain imaging in the same way. This is how cognitive scientist Sian Beilock studied hockey fans for her paper, "Sports Experience Enhances the Neural Processing of Action Language." She observed brain activity via functioning magnetic resonance imaging (fMRI). At Sapienza University of Rome, neuroscientist Salvatore Aglioti did a similar study with soccer fans, but used different brain activity scanning technology—transcranial magnetic stimulation (TMS).

To test levels of testosterone among fans of the winning and losing teams, behavioral scientist Paul Bernhardt showed up at Atlanta's Omni Coliseum armed with a bag of sterile vials. Working the pre-game crowd before a showdown of archrivals University of Georgia and Georgia Tech, he sought out spectators wearing the garb of either team, assuming they would be more representative of devoted fans, and asked them to spit into his vials, collecting saliva as he went. He later repeated his study for fans watching on TV by going to a sports bar showing soccer during the Brazil–Italy World Cup game to get more spit. A researcher in Lisbon conducted a similar spectator testosterone study but on a much different kind of sports fan: fish. Using aggressive Mozambique tilapia and setting up custom tanks with one-way mirrors, he took urine samples before and after fights from spectators—the other fish watching.

Urine figures surprisingly frequently in fan studies, sometimes in ways you would never expect. A graduate student in Dr. Wann's psychology program at Murray State got the idea that deeply invested fans might perceive odors differently based on team loyalty. So he soaked team jerseys in either a pleasant-smelling solution, like Febreze, or deer urine. They then had students who had been questioned to determine team identification smell each one and rate it. "It was interesting, but it didn't work. Turned out everyone just thought deer urine smelled terrible."

In a similar vein, Robin Dando, an associate professor in the Department of Food Science at Cornell University, handed out free ice cream samples at hockey games all season long to track whether fans' taste perceptions changed along with the final score. This time, unlike with smell, there was a correlation: the ice cream tasted better to victorious fans. The 2015 study found that food tasted better to people when the team they supported was winning. "When we looked at how they responded to these different flavors, in the games where they won, the flavors tasted sweeter and less sour, versus the opposite when they lost," Dando said. The researchers' best guess had to do with the neurotransmitter serotonin: you have more of it in your system when you're happy, which could influence taste, as there are serotonin receptors in our taste buds.

Sports fans have been demonstrated to merge their identity with that of their favorite teams—a deep investment that can lead them to make changes in their worldviews, as we will look at shortly. At the same time, fans' brains shut off the ignominy of defeat. There's an oft-cited corollary of these two habits, and many studies have shown that fans enjoying victory tend to claim a role, saying, "We won!" while they separate themselves from failure by saying, "They lost."

Sports psychology researcher Rick Grieve told me about how his doctoral team wanted to get data on exactly how passionate fans meld their identities with that of their favorite team, leading to a creative experiment. He and his PhD candidates staged the hallway to their offices with a seemingly random but actually carefully selected array of posters, still typical for a college hallway. These included an ad for the popular *Halo* video game, a Taylor Swift album promo, a poster for the latest movie in the Harry Potter series, and one sports poster, for the Nashville Predators, the geographically closest NHL team to Bowling Green, where the university is located, and the most popular one with locals. Without mentioning sports, they encouraged a large number of students to come by the office to answer questions for what sounded like an unrelated research project. Some survey questions assessed their self-described fandom for sports in general, and for hockey. They also asked each respondent if they could recall any of the posters they had walked past that day, and if so which ones. When the data was tabulated, the correlation between being a hockey fan and noticing that Predators poster was clear.

We were looking at how fans think they can influence
the outcomes of games. They can cheer, boo, curse, do
gestures, wave, pray, yell at refs. What we found was all
the ways they thought they could influence the outcome
were positively correlated. That is, if they wanted to try
to help their team in any way, they would do it in every
way they thought mattered. Hands clasped in prayer one
moment, cursing at the ref the next.
—**Dr. Dan Wann, as told to the author**

"The amount of sensory data in our environment is overwhelming," Dr. Grieve explained. "So we have a lot of filters
because there are so many inputs, but evolution keeps us
from filtering out the most important ones because we
need to be aware of those for survival." You might be hiking
in the woods and hear a lot of ambient natural noises—
wind rustling the leaves, birds chirping, water flowing, and
such—and mostly ignore it, but a branch snapping immediately behind you will get your attention in a hurry. "This
is also called the 'cocktail party effect,'" according to Dr.
Grieve. "You're in a crowded room, chatting, lots of conversations going on, and someone else says your name—you

overhear it and notice over everything else." This is a filtering phenomenon most of us have experienced—I know
I have. "Data suggests that highly identified fans have
adopted the importance of their team into their own identity, which is why their filter lets them notice that poster
and not the others," concluded Dr. Grieve. Science works
in mysterious ways, and for music fans, too: Taylor Swift,
whose followers are known as "Swifties," took home silver,
recalled by many of those identifying as music fans.

In *Blue Mind*, his water happiness treatise, Wallace J.
Nichols tries to explain how something we love, like water
(or sports) can become part of us, so ingrained in our identity as to cause neurochemical reactions in our brains without conscious effort when exposed to stimuli—even if,
unlike the NHL poster, we don't notice it. He describes an
experiment by psychologists at the University of Toronto
in which they built a simulated call center, and split volunteers into two groups. They instructed each on how to
make cold calls asking for donations to a charitable cause.
The instruction sheets were exactly the same, but for one
telling difference: one group got printed instructions that
included a photo of a woman runner crossing a finish line
and presumably winning a race, with no words or expla-
nation. The other one did not. Much to the researchers'
surprise, the group that saw the photo raised significantly

more money than their peers without a sports photo. They were so shocked by the outcome that they re-ran the experiment several more times with new volunteers; they always got the same results. "But here was what was so amazing about what happened," Nichols writes, "when the members of the groups that raised the most money were asked about the effect the picture of the victorious woman had on their solicitation, the same answer came back: "What picture?""

★ ★ ★ ★ ★ ★ ★ ★ ★ ★ ★ ★

A Houston Aeros hockey fan wrote, "Before every game I put my socks in the freezer for two hours and then wear them to the game." Perhaps just as interesting was his reason for this behavior, "This is what they do to the game pucks. I feel it gives us a slight advantage."
—Dr. Dan Wann, et al., "Examining the Superstitions of Sports Fans: Types of Superstitions, Perceptions of Impact, and Relationships with Team Identification"

★ ★ ★ ★ ★ ★ ★ ★ ★ ★ ★ ★

Deeper and longer in-person interviews are costly and time consuming, but sometimes they yield the most interesting results. Dr. Wann told me about when he and colleagues did a study of NASCAR fans, asking each to recall their recollection of the moment they heard of the death of legendary driver Dale Earnhardt, who was killed in a 2001 crash during the final lap of one the biggest motorsports races in the world, the Daytona 500. "These were one paragraph answers, and it took some people forty-five minutes to write it. Some just sat there. People started crying. Some were so soaked with tears we couldn't read them."

I asked Dr. Wann what was the most interesting study he had done in his decades of fan research, and without hesitation he started laughing. "We wanted to look at fan superstition, so we asked them to describe their sports-watching beliefs and superstitions. It was really fun, but it took us five years to code the responses, because they were all over the place and didn't easily fit into categories. What we did learn was that people really think what they do watching at home three hundred miles away affects the outcome of a game. People take this seriously and they feel guilty if they don't follow these superstitions and their team loses.

"A lot of it is apparel-related; what they wear when they watch. Some had lucky charms, including people—Mom can't watch with us because they always lose when she's here. We always lose when we go to the in-laws. Some was sex: one said, 'My wife has to call me Roger Clemens during sex the night before Clemens pitches.'"

Wann and eight colleagues, representing the psychology departments of eight universities, could find only two other existing studies on this topic, so they did their own. Nearly nineteen hundred people were interviewed and more than 40 percent reported at least one (and up to four) distinct superstitions. Many of these were extremely specific:

"Wear the jersey. If Pats are losing at halftime, take it off."

"If I'm sitting in a certain spot and the Astros are playing well, I stay there."

"During games, spouse and self must sit in winning spots (playoff games only)."

"If I eat grapefruit for breakfast, they win."

"Wish my friends good luck an odd number of times, not even, just odd."

"Stand during the last out of the bottom of the ninth inning—standing should occur only after there are two strikes on the batter."

"Always listen to every game on the radio. Even if the game's on TV we listen to the radio and just mute the TV."

"When the opposing team is on base I don't watch the pitch because I think I will jinx our pitcher and the other team will score runs."

"I have sex with nothing on but a jersey and one blue and one yellow sock on."

Because they wanted to differentiate between simple ritual (I wear the same shirt to games because I always have) and actual "superstitious behaviors believed to lead to or cause a specified outcome" (I wear the same shirt because then they win), they also asked why each respondent practiced the stated behavior. However, it warrants mention that some of the superstitions described below seem rather far-fetched. This may lead one to wonder whether the participant truly believed the action could impact the outcome of the event. Yet an examination of the "Why" responses provided strong validity for the superstitious nature of the information offered. For example . . . a University of Louisville football fan explained his food superstition ("I must have nachos and a bag of peanuts only to be followed by a hot dog") by stating "on notable occasions it has affected the outcome."

One Dallas Stars fan's game day food consumption process was vividly detailed. "At the old arena, every game I got in the Hebrew National Hot Dog line first. There, I bought a hot dog and a bottle of water. Then I got in the popcorn chicken line. I'd eat all but three to four bites of my hot dog in line, wrapped the rest up for my seat. At the first intermission, I got chocolate yogurt with M&Ms. At the new arena, I replaced both the hot dog and popcorn chicken with a chicken tender basket." Why this particular game time diet? "I want the Stars to win . . . and I'm doing my part."

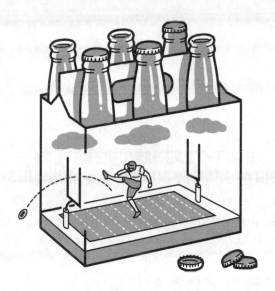

Wann's favorite? "One Notre Dame fan told us he had to drink three beers just before the start of every quarter." For those not keeping score at home, that's a lot of chugging and a twelve-pack per game. "One Notre Dame fan told us he had to read three Bible passages before each game. What was amazing to me is that it was the same fan. I have this image burned in my memory of this guy watching with a beer in one hand and a Bible in the other."

This particular line of investigation also revealed perhaps the best reason ever for not participating in sports psychology studies: "If I tell my 'game day rituals,' the team will almost undoubtedly lose."

POST-TRAUMATIC RECOVERY: HOW SPORTS HEALS COMMUNITIES

"You seem to have covered a lot of ground," said Dr. Kristie. "You've told me what Dr. Wann's favorite study was. So tell me, what was your favorite thing you learned during your research?"

It's a good question. Also a hard one, because there are so many benefits to being a fan. But to me, the most poignant and moving aspect is the power of fandom to heal—especially when life seems to be at its very worst.

While some psychologists study the everyday mental health of fans, other researchers have focused on how sports fandom helps us overcome and/or better deal with trauma, including personal loss, as well as communities devastated by disasters. Psychologists and professors Yuhei Inoue and Cody T. Havard of the University of Minnesota and University of Memphis, respectively, analyzed the effect of spectator sports on regions around the world hit by disasters over the eleven-year period between 2001 and 2011, a time frame that included major human-made events, most notably the 9/11 attacks in New York, and natural ones, such as Hurricane Katrina in 2005 and the 2011 Great East Japan Earthquake and ensuing tsunamis. They concluded that sports helped provide social support in post-disaster situations in eleven distinct ways, eight of which were tangible (fundraising, media attention to relief efforts, etc.) and three emotional, benefiting members of the affected communities.

This aspect of mental well-being may not be as easily measured as the other benefits, but major disasters have become so common that it is worth noting anything that can help. In just one year, 2013, Inoue and Havard documented a total of 330 natural hazards worldwide, which killed over twenty-one thousand people, affected 96.5 million individuals, and caused economic damages of roughly $120 billion. The same year also saw 158 human-made disasters, accounting for approximately six thousand deaths and $9 billion in economic damages.

"Have you ever been to the 9/11 Museum in New York?" I asked Dr. Kristie, who shook her head no. "I just visited for the first time this year and it was really intense for me."

The 9/11 Memorial Museum in lower Manhattan is a big, somber place, full of big, somber objects. Like the Twin Towers themselves, the scale makes visitors feel small as they stand before such oversized relics as a horribly crushed and burned fire truck, recovered engine parts, and ripped sections of fuselage from the aircrafts, along with the enormous pieces of twisted steel wreckage and pillars displayed throughout.

★ ★ ★ ★ ★ ★ ★ ★ ★ ★ ★ ★ ★

Tonight there will be a reason to sit next to strangers and feel connected by something other than fear and horror and sadness.
—Washington Post sportswriter Jennifer Frey's pre-game analysis of baseball's return following 9/11

★ ★ ★ ★ ★ ★ ★ ★ ★ ★ ★ ★ ★

The museum is set within the original subterranean foundation of the World Trade Center complex, and the exposed walls, rough concrete studded with steel ties, tower several floors overhead, adding to the dramatic scale. "Walking through the museum is like being transported back to the turmoil, destruction, and anguish of 9/11. Exhibits express the disbelief and heartache of New York and the nation," wrote the *Huffington Post*, accurately capturing the mood of the place. The opening review in the *New York Post* called the museum "as beautiful as it is horrific," adding that the exhibits are "a humanely crafted engine of catharsis."

I once worked in the World Trade Center, and as someone born and raised in New York, I'm old enough to remember when the Twin Towers first opened in 1973. They were the tallest buildings in the world and immediately transformed the Manhattan skyline. It was emotional for me to return, and the first time I did, the outdoor memorial was enough for one day. It took a second trip to the Ground Zero site for me to actually enter the museum, which I visited in the summer, peak tourist season. The line to get in was long and filled with foreign sightseers, most of whom seemed humbled by the solemnity of the place.

The experience begins before you even buy your ticket, as the museum is part of an eight-acre memorial complex, and the entrance is off the main memorial plaza where twin reflecting pools now occupy the footprints of the towers themselves. The pools, ringed by the names of the 2,983 victims etched in bronze, represent the voids that remain where the towers once stood. Once inside, I saw the eyes of more than a few visitors well up with tears. I could not hold back, either, not once I read the letter written by the then ten-year-old daughter of Captain Victor Saracini, pilot of hijacked United Airlines Flight 175, which was crashed into the South Tower that day. The letter shows the confusion of a child trying to come to grips with her loss and understand ungraspable concepts, like evil. It begins,

"Dear Derek Jeter, My name is Brielle Saracini. As you have heard, there was a horrible accident that involved the Twin Towers, there was a hijacking on a plane. Terrible people are in this world, but you and I both know that!"

While the single sheet of paper is one of the smallest objects displayed in the museum, it is also one of the most evocative. It was written to her favorite player, former New York Yankees star Derek Jeter, and was part of a nearly year-long special exhibition at the museum called "The Comeback Season: Sport After 9/11."

★ ★ ★ ★ ★ ★ ★ ★ ★ ★ ★ ★

After 9/11 there was a lot of chaos in this country, and people needed order. The ritual of sports is an important foundation in our lives and it provides that order we need.
—Hicks Wogan, National September 11 Museum
curator, as told to the author

★ ★ ★ ★ ★ ★ ★ ★ ★ ★ ★ ★

"What people look for in sports in a moment of crisis is security. You're going to games with people who are going through the same thing as you are. There's a kind of safety there. It feels good to have a sense of normalcy," said John Smith, a professor at Georgia Tech who teaches about sport history and the impact of sports on society. "Sports really are the most visible place where people can come together outside of churches. And let's face it, arenas are bigger than most churches. I can think of no other place where so many people come out to show their support for people who are grieving, who have lost something, who are going through tragedy."

The exhibit opened with a facsimile of the exterior of Wrigley Field, baseball's second oldest stadium, adorned on 9/11 with a huge sign informing visitors that today's game was canceled—as was every other major professional sporting event in the nation. It was the first time since the death of President Franklin Delano Roosevelt that Major League Baseball canceled all its games. Stadiums would remain dark for over a week. New York Jets quarterback Vinny Testaverde visited workers at Ground Zero and told his coach and teammates that if the league decided to go ahead with the games that weekend, they could go ahead without him, and he was immediately backed by his teammates and coach Herm Edwards, who decided that if forced to play, they would forfeit. They didn't have to, and on September 13, NFL Commissioner Paul Tagliabue said, "At a certain point, playing our games can contribute to the healing process. Just not at this time."

"It was never a question of if sports would resume as normal, the big question was when," said Hicks Wogan, assistant director of exhibition development for the National September 11 Memorial & Museum (its official name), who curated the objects in the sports exhibit and wrote the supporting display text.

When the games did come back, they did so with a vengeance, and they certainly contributed to the healing process as Tagliabue had predicted. Most memorable was the Atlanta Braves visiting the New York Mets at Shea Stadium, the first major sports event played in New York City since the attacks. "I was at that game," recalled Dr. Soumi Eachempati, an emergency surgeon and professor who was then director of the Surgical Intensive Care Unit at New York-Presbyterian/Weill Cornell Medical Center. "It was crazy. Marc Anthony sang the national anthem and you could have heard a pin drop, it was so serious. But by the seventh inning, when Liza Minnelli sang 'New York, New York,' everyone was into the game. Everyone was waving American flags." Dr. Eachempati is a rabid sports fan, and he also attended the home Yankees games in the World Series that year, when President Bush famously threw a perfect strike as the opening pitch and Derek Jeter hit a dramatic walk-off home run. "The rest of the games that year did so much to bring people back together."

> Sports gives us our sense of community
> in times of grief. It's like our collective couch,
> helping to soothe our national pain.
> **—Associated Press writer Paul Newberry's
> commentary "It's Time for Sports to
> Help Us Heal Again"**

Matthew Andrews, a sports-centric history professor at the University of North Carolina, was also at the World Series. "I was not a big George W. Bush guy at all, but when he was throwing out the ball for Game Three in the 2001 World Series, I was rooting for him to throw a strike, and it actually felt meaningful that it was a strike in some ridiculous way," Andrews told me. "If it was high and outside it would have been like 'Oh my God, we can't do anything right in this country.' It was a strike, right down the middle, and I show it in my class, and I can see that same feeling in my students' eyes."

Now an adult, Brielle Saracini, who wrote the letter to Jeter as a ten-year-old, narrated a short film for the museum exhibit in which she notes that the Yankee wins in the Bronx were so memorable that most people forget that they ultimately lost the World Series. But that hardly matters because they won at home.

For the Mets–Braves game, most of the nation—with the possible exception of Braves fans—were rooting for New York, who came from behind on the fairy tale eighth-inning, game-winning home run, absolutely crushed by catcher Mike Piazza, who played in a helmet emblazoned with the FDNY logo. After the game, Piazza would observe, "People want to find refuge in sports, especially in baseball, want to find comfort in a crowd, being around other people. Maybe that has a tendency to ease the pain even if it's just a little bit."

Howie Rose, the Mets' veteran radio voice, was doing TV coverage that day, and he recalled how the real impact of the moment became apparent a minute after the home run, when Piazza reemerged from the dugout for a bow. Rose saw a group of firemen who had been invited to the game as guests standing in their dress uniforms, smiling and laughing and reveling in the movement. "And I just immediately wondered: 'What have the last ten days been like for those guys? They lost friends, colleagues, God forbid other family members. And now they look like *this*. Baseball did that for them.'"

Years later, after retiring, Braves star Chipper Jones told *Sports Illustrated*:

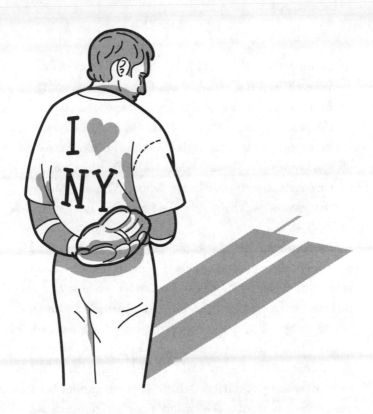

Those fans who showed up that night, they just wanted to see some baseball. They didn't hate the Atlanta Braves. They just wanted to see two good baseball teams and forget about their troubles for a few hours ... There was no way in hell we were going to win that game. I've had maybe ten, fifteen, or twenty instances in my career where I've had a premonition. I was playing leftfield that night. When Mike Piazza walked up, I knew he was going to hit a home run. I said to myself before the pitch, the roof is going to come off this place, if he hits a home run right here. Sure enough, he took Steve Karsay deep . . . Usually when someone hits a home run against you, your heart drops. When he hit it that night, I was happy for the fans. They needed it.

Professor Andrews loves playing devil's advocate and is generally full of contrarian examples for any argument. I asked him if the positive power of sports to help communities after trauma was supported by historical evidence. "I like to be a bit of the fly in the ointment, but here's where I think the answer unequivocally is yes. Sports has absolutely played that role and it's because of the primacy of sports, the popularity. I think without a doubt these are really important places where people can just be emotional, talk about feelings. After September 11, baseball stadiums seemed to be places where people could talk about healing and coming together, where Red Sox fans sang 'New York, New York' and Pittsburgh fans wore 'I LOVE NY' pins. I thought that was pretty special. Where did that happen, where else can it happen other than at sporting events?"

> That game was the moment when we went
> from being citizens full of rage and sorrow
> and anger to being fans again, when it was
> okay to clap again, and to laugh and smile.
> **—Denver sports fan Taylor Shields,**
> **as told to the author**

Despite having lived and breathed this material for the past couple of years, I still get teary when I reflect on the power of sports after 9/11, so I shared the story of Carol Gies with Dr. Kristie. Carol is the widow of New York City Fire Department Lieutenant Ronnie E. Gies, one of the heroes and first responders killed in the World Trade Center attack.

Ten days later, on September 21, Gies and her three sons attended that first game between the Mets and the Braves at Shea Stadium, where fans were greeted with a never-before-seen level of ballpark security, an ominous reminder of the recent events. As many people I spoke to told me, New York City needed the win and Mike Piazza gave it to them. His home run has become one of the most iconic moments in baseball history.

"Going to the game was very difficult. My husband and all of us were huge Mets fans, Ronnie coached our sons in Little League, and we just felt like Shea was the place we had to be," Gies recalled later. "When that ball went over the wall, I saw my children smile for the first time since they lost their dad. 9/11 went away for that one split second, and to see my children excited and smiling, I was like 'You know what, we're going to do this, we're going to get through it.'" After the game, Gies and her sons were escorted to the dugout by police and got to meet Piazza and the rest of the team. Twelve years later, when the Mets inducted Piazza into the team's Hall of Fame, Gies was there, to meet the star catcher in person once again. "I wouldn't miss this day for the world. None of us will ever forget what this man did to help our family." Many witnesses did not forget: nearly two decades later, Mets fan Patrick Barry, a member of the US Army's elite Special Forces and instructor in the highest-tier Ranger training program, would tell an *Outside Magazine* rewriter that Piazza's blast was "the most important swing of my life."

As a mother herself, Dr. Kristie could relate, and I could see that she was especially moved. But 9/11 was no anomaly; rather, it was one of many examples of sports helping communities through their darkest hours. I asked Dr. Kristie if she would allow me one more example. She was willing to indulge me, and I told her about my recent trip to Las Vegas, where one of the many people I spoke to was Nick Robone.

"I was shot in the chest," Robone told me in as level a voice and as matter-of-factly as anyone could possibly say such a thing. "I was at the concert that night, I was shot, and fortunately I'm still here to talk about it."

He is talking about the Route 91 Harvest music festival, an annual country music event featuring multiple bands that, on October 1, 2017, was headlined by Jason Aldean and held outdoors at an open-air venue on the other side of Las Vegas Boulevard, aka "The Strip," across from the huge Mandalay Bay Resort and Casino complex. The tragedy that unfolded during the concert is historically known as the 2017 Las Vegas Shooting, but to locals, where it is treated as the city's own 9/11, it is referred to as One October—or in the circumspect way such things are discussed in hushed tones, The Event, The Tragedy, The Nightmare, or simply The Concert.

Whatever you call it, that night was the worst mass shooting in American history, when deranged Nevada resident Stephen Paddock broke the glass in the window of his thirty-second-floor suite in Mandalay Bay and began firing on the crowd below, right near Las Vegas Boulevard. Chaos and carnage ensued as concert-goers had no idea where the shots were coming from or who was firing them. Many thought the venue had been invaded by multiple attackers, causing people to remain in place and hide under tables and whatever cover was available as Paddock continued firing down at them. Security fences trapped many panicked fans. Some gates were torn down and people were trampled and confused and terrified as they fled in all directions, crushed up against barriers. Police were initially just as confused about where the shots were coming from, and for a full ten minutes, which seemed like hours to those in the crowd, Paddock continued firing and reloading from his personal arsenal, which included fourteen semi-automatic assault rifles, most of which had been modified to fire at a fully automatic pace. He averaged nearly two shots per second, and in those roughly six hundred seconds of terror, fired over 1,100 bullets.

For ten long minutes, the Las Vegas Strip, one of the world's most popular tourist sites, was turned into a killing zone, and by the time Paddock took his own life as police approached his door, he had murdered 58, shot another 422, and more than 400 others were injured in the pandemonium. Several area hospitals saw their emergency rooms and trauma wards overrun with shooting victims, one of whom was Nick Robone.

Robone is the associate head coach of the men's hockey team at the University of Nevada Las Vegas (UNLV). Shot in the chest with a high-powered assault rifle, a gun specifically designed to cause the maximum possible damage,

Robone knows he is lucky to be alive. Remarkably, he has fully recovered physically, and when I spoke to him ten months after the attack, he was skating with his team again. He spent six days in the intensive care unit, and another four in a "regular" room at the hospital. He was finally released, and just two days later, on October 12, he returned to the Strip, and once again plunged into the crowds adjacent to Mandalay Bay, this time to attend his very first Golden Knights NHL game.

Some of the greatest moments in sports are the Cinderella stories, the remarkable upsets, the unexpected seasons—these are the scenarios that often move spectators the most. But few tales seem more likely to have been scripted by Hollywood than the real-life first season of the Golden Knights—and the remarkable benefits it brought fans and the more than two million residents of Las Vegas.

"It's as improbable as ice in the desert," said the anchors of *CBS This Morning*. "A year ago the Las Vegas Golden Knights didn't even exist. Their roster is full of players that, shall we say, were not priorities for other clubs. Then something extraordinary happened—this team no one expected to win kept winning."

Regardless of the sport, the debuts of expansion teams, those created out of whole cloth, are notoriously poor performances. After all, sports fans hear their teams talk all the time about multi-year plans or rebuilding seasons while a new team has no such opportunity—and typically no star players or developmental pipeline. When the New York Mets were let loose upon the baseball public in 1962, they posted the worst record in modern history, a still untouchably terrible 40–120 season that saw them finish more than sixty games out of first place. In fact, expansion teams do so poorly that it was widely considered a "miracle" when the Mets won their first World Series "just" seven years later. So for the Knights to be playing in the fifth game of the Stanley Cup Finals for the season championship just eighteen months after unveiling their name and logo is uncharted territory. The Knights began the season as 500–1 longshots in the Las Vegas sports betting books—and that's probably generous with home-field advantage and local fan betting support.

The Knights' debut season also saw another sports history first—they retired a jersey number no player had ever worn. It was fifty-eight, the death toll of One October. The new team opened its inaugural season at home in a city that was not known for hockey fans and had no major professional sports teams, a city still numb and reeling from a tragedy so large that almost no one was untouched. For a metropolis of two million and a major tourist destination, Las Vegas has a remarkably small-town feel among the locals. "Everyone was affected," said Brian Killingsworth, chief marketing officer and senior vice president for the Golden Knights. "Whether it was two or three degrees of separation, you knew someone who was there. We actually had a couple of people in our organization at the concert, and our players were down on the Strip at that time. For us it hit home personally."

It was in this dark mood, just nine days after the shooting, that the Golden Knights took to their home ice for the first time. They won. Then they won again. When they won for the third time they became the first expansion team in NHL history to do so. They won eight of their first nine games, also a record. They would never leave first place for the rest of the season, and Las Vegans took to the team like no fans ever. Los Angeles Dodgers team historian Mark Langill described the personal and community healing power of fandom to me as "sports medicine," and the Knights were the perfect prescription for what ailed the city. They broke records at the cash register, too, selling more merchandise than any team in the league. Well after the first season, when I returned to Vegas to interview team executives, politicians, victims, and survivors, I couldn't help but notice that just about every car in the city seemed to sport a Golden Knights sticker. Knights logos were on shirts and hats and houses, and in lights on buildings on game days. They were everywhere.

I asked local acquaintances if they knew anyone who had been at the concert and would talk to me about it, which led me to Nick Robone and Jessica Duran. "I got split up from my friends, it was the ultimate chaos. I was running for my life," Duran told me. She is a marketing manager for the liquor division of global luxury goods giant Louis Vuitton Möet Hennessy (LVMH) and she was hosting a VIP suite in a temporary outdoor structure on the concert grounds when shots shattered the windows and sent her scrambling for cover. She fled out the back of the suite scaffolding, jumping to the ground and running out through a section of fence that quick-thinking mechanics had ripped down with a chain and truck, finally running onto the still-active runway of the abutting private jet terminal, where she was happy to be "apprehended" by police who didn't yet fully realize what was going on. Several of her friends were shot. "There was a period of time after that when I just wouldn't leave the house. It was a little too traumatic."

Duran was already having a bad year—her mom had just died two months earlier—and now she sought professional help. "I was talking to my therapist about the healing process, what do you do now, how do you move forward from here, and I remember telling her that I had been invited to a hockey game." Her therapist urged her to think about it carefully and consider whether she really wanted to be in a crowd situation like that, back on the Strip, after what she has just experienced. Duran thought about it and decided that, no, she did not. So she stayed home. Lots of her friends had season tickets and kept inviting her, then after five or six games, she gave in. "I felt life does go on, you have to move on at some point, and there was this sense that all these amazing things were happening around the Knights. I thought, 'Okay, this is something I can do. I said, why not, let's do it.'

"It was amazing. I've been a huge sports fan all my life, baseball, college basketball, but I'd never watched a hockey game. I didn't know the rules, and it's complicated. But it all just clicked for me and I thought, 'You're supposed to be here, you're supposed to be part of this, get out of this crazy rut, don't be scared of crowds and of what could happen. You need to take control of your life.' That all happened the first game, it was very emotional for me."

★ ★ ★ ★ ★ ★ ★ ★ ★ ★ ★

**We had just been brought to our knees by
this horrible, diabolical tragedy. The pain was so deep,
it was seared into us all. Then for the Golden Knights
to have that season and start the healing process,
the timing was incredible.
—Las Vegas Mayor Carolyn Goodman,
as told to the author**

★ ★ ★ ★ ★ ★ ★ ★ ★ ★ ★

There are many striking elements to the healing story of the Knights, and one is the fact that so many people like Duran, who knew nothing about hockey and had never seen a game, are now passionate devotees. Duran

has Golden Knights T-shirts, hats, golf shirts, and sometimes takes her dad to games, gifting him his own logo gear.
After dipping her toe in, she would return to the T-Mobile
Arena about fifty more times that season. "From that first
moment, I went to every single game I could get tickets
to, and I traveled to LA for the first round of the playoffs
against the Kings. I have a lot of friends with season tickets, but when they weren't available I just bought them on
StubHub because it was something I really wanted to be
part of." When they were out of town she watched on TV—
there were, and still are, huge Knights viewing parties for
every game all over Vegas—in bars, in the casinos, and even
at the team's training facility in suburban Summerlin, some
of which draw thousands of fans. Thousands also routinely
show up just to watch practices, and while they keep some
game seats open for out-of-town guests, there are more
than enough season ticket holders and would-be season
ticket holders on the waitlist—now closed—to easily fill
the arena every night without a single walk-in.

"We wanted to win, we needed to win, for the city and
everyone here," said Knights star Deryk Engelland (Duran's
favorite player). The Knights opted to go with no official
captain, but it was Engelland who addressed the opening-
day crowd, speaking about the elephant in the arena, the
nation's worst mass shooting. "Like all of you," he said
before the game, "I'm proud to call Las Vegas home. To

the families and friends of the victims, know that we'll do everything we can to help you and our city heal."

And they did. Not just by winning or by hosting survivors, heroes, and first responders at every game, all season, and not just with a somber fifty-eight seconds of silence before the puck drops at each game. But by going out into the community, visiting victims in hospitals, showing up at station houses to shake hands with firefighters, skating with the youth groups they host for free at their own rink, and being seemingly at all places all the time, on and off the ice. "We went down to the players and offered them the chance go out and visit police, firemen, hospitals, and to a man they all volunteered and went out, during the week of our home opener," Knights SVP Killingsworth told me. "They went to the blood banks to thank people for giving blood." Everyone I talked to in Las Vegas, without exception, from the mayor to casino executives to Uber drivers to bartenders, praised the Knights as an absolutely necessary healing balm for their city.

Players visited college coach Robone in the hospital after he was shot. I asked him how important he thought the Knights were in terms of helping him and the city in which he had been born and raised. "One hundred percent. Whether emotionally or physically, they helped me personally in several ways. And the city really needed a distraction, something else to think about. A lot of people were hurting, really struggling to cope. It gave the city something to cheer for again. And it did more than that. People talked to neighbors they had never talked to before. People talked to strangers. I think they would have had a big positive impact on the city minus One October, and even without the shooting I think for sure they would have greatly helped give us a sense of community, but it was like a perfect storm."

The Knights' Killingsworth had previously worked for teams in Major League Baseball, and one of the first things he did after the shooting was call his former baseball colleagues at the Boston Red Sox for advice. "Sports is a great unifier, and my friends in Boston immediately identified with our tragedy because they had been through it, too. I asked how they had dealt with the Boston Marathon bombing."

Boston's response to that tragedy in April 2013 has become baseball legend. As with 9/11, it began with the postponement of the next game. Then the players replaced the words Red Sox on their jerseys with Boston. They brought out survivors to throw first pitches and honored first responders and families of victims. As the *Athletic* put it, "For the next five days, the city was on edge and even on lockdown. Not until Friday night, when the terrorist Dzhokhar Tsarnaev was apprehended after he and his brother engaged law enforcement in an extensive manhunt, was the city able to breathe again. During that week and the rest of that season, the Red Sox became a symbol of the city's resilience, their traditional serifed B incorporating

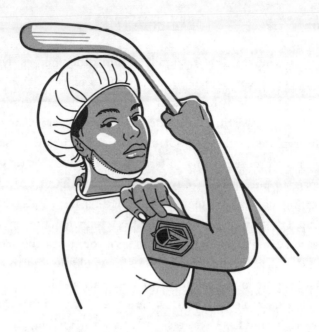

itself in the Boston Strong logo. They visited hospitals, they honored victims, and they won the World Series."

Red Sox catcher David Ross was one of many players who visited victims in hospitals following the bombing. "I felt such a responsibility from then on out—I think everybody did—that we were playing for more than just our organization. We were playing for those people in those beds, for those doctors and nurses and the city, trying to get them something positive to cling onto that year."

At the first Las Vegas Knights game, instead of the traditional introduction of the players, the team honored doctors, nurses, first responders, and other heroes, who were each accompanied onto the ice by a player. "It wasn't about the Golden Knights, it was about the community," said Killingsworth. All the ads in the arena were removed and replaced with #VegasStrong signs. T-shirts were sold with the proceeds going to families of victims. "As we got closer to our opener we realized the game had to be this healing moment. We mourned the victims, but we also celebrated the first responders." Months later, when the regular season came to an end, the team sponsored a tattoo artist on the plaza outside the arena, who would do a tattoo of the Knights logo—a real, permanent tattoo—in exchange for a charitable donation. During the playoffs more than one thousand Las Vegas residents took the lifelong plunge. As he recalled, "One of my favorite things I heard was a fan interviewed who said, 'The Golden Knights gave Las Vegas a soul.'"

SPORTS AND SPIRITUAL HEALING

*K*illingsworth talked about souls, Duran about karma and destiny, and comparisons of sports and religion are made frequently. Both involve heavy doses of faith, prayer, coming together, and healing, and it's no coincidence that important athletic venues, from Yankee Stadium to the Indianapolis Motor Speedway, are often described as temples of their respective sports. So I asked Randall Balmer, a priest, distinguished professor of religion at Dartmouth College, and lifelong diehard Detroit Lions fan, about this connection.

"I think it's overtaken religion," he said of sports fandom. "It takes you out of yourself a little bit, and that's a good thing." As for the role of sports in the spiritual healing of communities, Balmer is a big believer. "I've thought about this a great deal because I grew up as a Detroit Tigers fan, and when they won the 1968 World Series, that was the year after the Detroit riot." He refers to the bloodiest of more than a hundred and fifty race riots across the nation in what has been called "The Long Hot Summer of 1967." It resulted in more than forty deaths and the destruction of approximately two thousand buildings in the city. Michigan's governor eventually called in the National Guard and President Lyndon Johnson sent in two US Army units, including the famed 101st Airborne. A year later the Tigers won it all. "It was a moment of healing, a balm at that much-needed time. I remember it very clearly. It helped heal a very troubled city."

In 2017, on the fiftieth anniversary of the riot, sports columnist Pat Caputo reflected on the power of sports at the worst moments in our lives: "Even during the most polarizing of times, those in the suburbs crossed Eight Mile continually to see the Tigers and the Red Wings . . . I'm not suggesting the '68 Tigers healed Detroit's wounds, but they were a much-needed tourniquet that greatly helped control profuse bleeding . . . [T]he timing of their arrival was perfectly scripted." Former *New York Times* and *Detroit Free Press* sports reporter Joe Lapointe was a teenage usher at Tiger Stadium during the 1968 season. Lapointe described the victory as a big one for an ailing Detroit and said, "It's one of our treasured municipal myths. And I use the word myths in the highest sense . . . as a traditional story of supernatural heroes and great things happening that are hard to explain. As sort of a magic story."

Thanks to the infamy of 9/11, One October, the Boston Marathon Bombing, and other attacks, the healing power of sports in the face of violence has been amply demonstrated. But natural disasters are more common and often more destructive than human-made ones, and here, too, fandom plays a powerful and comforting role. The 9/11 Museum "Comeback Season" curator Hicks Wogan was living in New Orleans in 2005, and he told me how the Saints' Super Bowl win greatly helped the city's battered morale after Hurricane Katrina. Another example occurred in 2018 as Category Five Hurricane Lane slammed into the Hawaiian Islands, causing fires, sending residents to emergency shelters, and dropping more than forty inches of rain on parts of the Big Island, the hearts and minds of many residents were pleasantly distracted by activities more than five thousand miles away. In Williamsport, Pennsylvania, the state's all-star lineup of youth baseball players—the "Boys of the 808," the state's sole area code—were battling for the top spot at the Little League World Series.

On the night before the US championship final, the team posted a video of support for those back home, ending with, "Dear Hawaii, while you are thinking of them, they are thinking of you." As the *Honolulu Star-Advertiser* noted, "The team's run . . . continues to captivate the state despite the massive threat of Lane." *CBS Sports* wrote, "As

Hurricane Lane approaches, Hawaii is playing for more than a trophy. As the massive threat of Hurricane Lane looms over Hawaii, the state can turn to an unlikely source for solace: The group of preteens representing Hawaii at the Little League World Series."

Hawaii won, and in dominating statement fashion, went undefeated throughout the entire tournament, winning the last three games to clinch the US and then World Championships (against Korea) with a trio of consecutive shutouts. In an interview afterward, the team's manager, Gerald Oda, explained that, "What they're going through is very difficult—we've been there—all of us have been there when these storms have come. And it can be chaotic, it's a lot of stress. But we told the kids that . . . this is our opportunity to really give back. Because we know that there's a lot of people at home watching the game. And we said that if anything, for them to watch us, we can give them hope. They can take their mind off. And that's what we hope it did."

Psychology professors Yuhei Inoue and Cody T. Havard have tracked the positive effects of sports on natural and human-made disasters. But nothing they had studied compared to the global impact the 2020 coronavirus pandemic had, infecting millions, killing hundreds of thousands, shutting down or severely impacting the economies of every nation. During the pandemic, I asked Dr. Havard about how sports would figure into our long-term recovery. He felt that sports would again be able to play a healing role after coronavirus.

"People use their love of sports to cope with natural disasters. Sports create a diversion, and also watching sports or being emotionally invested in the outcomes allows someone to distance from their realities and feel involved in something other than their daily lives." However, he explained that the healing properties of fandom were not limited to massive disasters and global epidemics. It could also apply to individual suffering: "Even a diversion of a couple or few hours can help someone going through tragedy."

The late Michelle Musler used sports to help her through personal trauma. She told the *New York Times* how she came to be one of basketball's most devoted fans: "My ex-husband ran away with the lady next door and I didn't seem to fit into suburbia anymore." She had occasionally gotten free tickets from her company for Knicks games and after her husband left her she turned to the team in a big way—she upgraded to season tickets, and over the next twenty-seven years missed only a handful of games, planning her business travel around the team's schedule, even flying back from a work trip in Hong Kong to make a game. "The Knicks gave me a purpose, something to do, a place to go. As a fan, I guess, there is a sense of belonging. That you are a part of something,"

SPORTS HEALS

As Dr. Kristie and I talked about Michelle Musler's experience and those of others who embraced fandom's welcome, we got on the topic of the power of positive thinking. I asked if as a physician she believed that the mind could help heal the body?

"Personally, yes, I do," she replied. "There is increasing research that mindfulness and meditation, which were once seen as New Age-y, have a role in modern medicine. Positivity certainly can't hurt."

During my own research I heard about many stories of individuals who believed they had harnessed their love of sports to fight disease or overcome injury, but I wanted to talk to someone who had gone through this firsthand. I asked Kasey Storey, my former student at Dartmouth, where she was getting her master's in creative writing, who had agreed to be my research assistant for this book, to help me with the search. Her immediate response: "You should talk to my mom."

★ ★ ★ ★ ★ ★ ★ ★ ★ ★ ★ ★ ★

**When you watch athletes, and see what the
human body is capable of, you're more inspired to do
what you can for your own body. It was a scary, awful,
painful time, and having something for you, whatever
it is, is really helpful. For me, it's the Broncos.**
—Cancer survivor Kelly Storey

★ ★ ★ ★ ★ ★ ★ ★ ★ ★ ★ ★ ★

"I can't remember ever not being a Broncos fan," Kasey's
mother, Kelly Storey, told me. She is also a self-declared
"huge" fan of Rockies baseball, a hockey lover, fantasy
league enthusiast, and serious sports fan through and
through, but like so many people from the Mile High State,
the Broncos come first.

"Sports were really important to me and my dad his
whole life. He got Wegener's disease, an autoimmune disor-
der, and lost his hearing when I was five. I watched a lot of
baseball with Dad; he taught me how to score. It was really
important to my dad to do those things we could still do
together even though he was deaf, and when he was sick
and couldn't do much physically, it was very important
bonding going to baseball games and watching football.
The father/daughter bonding we had was so important, it
turned me into a sports fan forever. We watched football

together every Sunday. I was obsessed with it; my dad was the only one who even remotely loved it as much as I did. I still vividly remember the day I turned eighteen and was old enough to drink 3.2 percent beer. My dad and I sat on the couch that Sunday and had our first drink together while we watched the game. It's one of those memories that I'll never forget."

Kelly Storey believes that her father's fandom helped him deal with his Wegener's disease, and combat his physical decline. It may not have given him any more time, but he made the time he had left much better. Years later she would put this lesson to good use and rely on her love of football to battle her own bout with mortality.

She realized something was wrong in 1997, after her beloved Broncos got off to an unusually successful 6–0 start. She could literally feel it in her bones—Broncos fans have a tradition of bringing down the "Rocky Mountain Thunder" at home games to befuddle opponents. This is a clamor that comes from jumping up and down on the metal stands, or stomping their feet on the metal floor. But when the thirty-two-year-old Storey did it, something felt wrong, something in her leg.

She had bone cancer. After learning that she needed surgery on her leg, and quickly, Kelly was able to attend just one more game the following Sunday, and she defiantly stomped even harder. "My husband had bought me

the tickets as a birthday present. The Broncos were playing the Seattle Seahawks at home on my actual birthday,
November second. I had surgery scheduled and remember
thinking about that tumor in my leg, and I wasn't sure if I
was ever going be able to cheer like this again."

Twenty years and numerous surgeries later, she still
favors orange and blue, a limited palette that covers almost
her entire closet from pajamas to winter coats. Her house
is marked by a handcrafted Broncos yard ornament, her
door by a giant Broncos helmet decal on the glass. In the
foyer, guests are greeted by a stained-glass Broncos logo, a
Broncos birdhouse, and an autographed Peyton Manning
helmet (his signed jersey is displayed in another room).
Her kitchen cupboards hold Super Bowl 50 napkins and
Broncos tumbler glasses. But if there has been one magi-
cal talisman in the Storey home over all these years, it was
the flood-damaged, life-sized cardboard John Elway cutout,
once displayed at a Best Buy store advertising DirecTV, a
weathered but still standing survivor, like Kelly Storey
herself.

For the seven weeks following her surgery, the Broncos
fought to stay in the hunt for their elusive first-ever Super
Bowl championship, and an inspired Kelly fought, too. At
first she spent games on the couch in a cast that ran from
the base of her toes to the top of her hip, as the cardboard
Elway, a gift from an understanding uncle, stood vigil over

her recovery. On the TV, and on the field, the real John Elway won game after game, and on January 11, 1998, the Denver Broncos punched their ticket to the Super Bowl.

When they met the Green Bay Packers for the championship in San Diego on January 25, Kelly was still on the couch, still in the cast, but now she was more mobile, using crutches. As she cheered, the Broncos won their first-ever Super Bowl, 31–24.

"We had to overcome so much adversity as a team, we had to make the wild card game and overcome our losses," she recalled. At the same time, she began physical therapy, and her recovery included tough treadmill sessions, coached by the cardboard Elway, positioned in front of the machine for inspiration. She won't go quite so far as to claim the Broncos were entirely responsible for her recovery, but being a fan helped her immeasurably. "It would have been much, much harder without football. I wanted to sack this disease."

For her comeback season in 1998, when she traded her cast for a brace, and a cane for crutches, the Storeys decided to splurge on their first two season tickets. Real John Elway announced he would play only one more season, and cardboard John Elway continued to cheer Kelly on as she plodded through physical therapy and treadmill workouts. By the time the Broncos went deep in the playoffs for the second straight year, she was not only able to attend the home games, she once again called down the Rocky Mountain Thunder. "The '98–'99 season we just seemed so dominant, so unstoppable. It seemed like we were destined for success. It was just so amazing after winning last year in spite of some major struggles." It is sometimes hard to tell when she's talking about the Broncos' performance or her own trials and tribulations, because to her they are forever intertwined. A year after ending a franchise Super Bowl drought that had gone on since before she was born, the Broncos won again, besting the Atlanta Falcons 34–19 in Miami for Super Bowl XXXIII on January 31, 1999. Two weeks later, Kelly was walking without a cane, cancer-free.

Kelly Storey leveraged her passion as a sports fan into a health tool, but she was not the only fan battling cancer to rely on her team for inspiration. There are many similar stories, involving both adults and children, in just about every sport. In fact, Storey is not even close to being unique as a woman Broncos fan going through this experience— there have been so many that the team saluted them with its "Fight Like A Bronco" anti-cancer campaign. One was Shelly Gibbons, who in the fall of 2013, as football season was starting and new Broncos quarterback Peyton Manning was setting more records, learned that she had Stage IV breast cancer. She would later say that following the team's quest for the Super Bowl kept her sane and allowed her to feel she was living a normal life. For every visit to the hospital for rounds of drug injections, she wore her favorite "chemo outfit," an old number 7 John Elway jersey, to remind her not to give up. Fittingly for both Storey and Gibbons, their role model was famous for never giving up, and Elway is so synonymous with miraculous last-minute, come-from-behind victories that there have been numerous articles written ranking his five or ten best fourth-quarter career comebacks. After all, he had thirty-one such games where he snatched victory from the jaws of defeat in the final period—more than a fifth of his career wins—along with forty game-winning drives, football's equivalent of the walk-off home run. He is fifth in NFL history for fourth quarter comebacks, and Peyton Manning, who replaced him as the Broncos quarterback, is number one. It may seem melodramatic to some to say that the Broncos saved Shelley Gibbons. But not to her. As she explained, "They absolutely kept me fighting, too."

Science writer Eric Simons described the case of Raiders super-fan Steve Winfield:

> He'd been diagnosed with colon cancer a few years earlier, and now he'd run out of options. He'd had surgery. He'd tried chemo . . . Finally in the fall of 2002 he'd gone to Hawaii to try one more New Age type healing treatment. Somewhere on that trip, his brother Ken went out to visit, and everyone

realized that nothing was going to work. There were no more options. Steve started to change then, Ken says, in an odd way. Instead of that constant restlessness, he finally settled into his identity. He was a Raiders fan, and he was going to die as one . . . Steve started to focus on a goal. The Raiders were going to make it to the Super Bowl and he was going to make it with them. Vegas liked the Raiders' odds of playing into February, but the doctor didn't like Steve's. So he leaned on the Raiders and he defied the doctors. When the regular season ended in January, the Raiders were the top seed in the AFC playoffs and Steve had already lived for a few months past his expiration date . . . it seemed like the Raiders' success was keeping Stevie alive, a kind of literal demonstration of self-expansion theory.

The Raiders reached the Super Bowl, but they lost, and a few hours later Winfield slipped into a coma and died. His brother Ken said, "He really was at peace. The Raiders brought him to a point where, once the Super Bowl was over, he was okay to pass away."

I spoke about Steve with Dr. Philip Anton, an associate professor of exercise physiology at Southern Illinois University, who sees a lot of cancer survivors firsthand as the founder and program director of the Strong Survivor

Exercise and Nutrition Program for Cancer Survivors and Caregivers. "I had a patient who was a big Michigan fan and he got diagnosed with cancer just before they made their run to the Final Four. He used that as both his motivation to recover and as distraction from the negatives of the disease. I think it definitely helped, it made a real difference, and I've seen and heard about lots of similar cases."

"Any of us who take care of kids who have these conditions can reel off anecdote after anecdote about this effect, but it's nice to see real numbers back that up," Doug Scothorn, MD, PhD, told me. Dr. Scothorn is a Pediatric Hematologist/Oncologist at Mission Hospital in Asheville, North Carolina, a professor at the UNC School of Medicine, and serves on the national medical advisory board for the Make-A-Wish Foundation.

SPORTS WISHES DO COME TRUE

*N*ow, finally, I was speaking Dr. Kristie's language: medicine.

Because he sees almost exclusively children with cancer, Dr. Scothorn also sees a lot of kids who end up getting wishes granted by the Make-A-Wish Foundation, a high-profile non-profit organization that arranges dream experiences, known as "wishes," for children with life-threatening medical conditions. He believes that these wishes provide concrete medical benefits to the children, and according to Make-A-Wish America, 74 percent of parents later said the wish marked a turning point in their child's response to treatment. Make-A-Wish has over sixty chapters around the country and is active in more than forty other countries. Sports-related wishes are second only to a trip to Disney in requests the group receives. Thousands are granted every year, from meeting sports heroes to attending big events like the World Series to driving around racetracks in a NASCAR car with a beloved driver.

"As far as sports and Make-A-Wish, it is always one of our most popular things. We have kids who want to be a member of a sports team for a day, and we've had kids who want to meet a particular athlete. To go to the Super Bowl is a really popular wish," said Casey Thompson of the national office of Make-A-Wish America in Phoenix. Some athletes are so devoted to the cause that they have granted hundreds of wishes over the years.

I called Dr. Scothorn because I had heard so many anecdotes about sports fandom having a meaningful impact on people's health, and I wanted to know if there was more concrete scientific evidence. It is important to realize that his data covers all wishes, not just sports, but sports are responsible for a substantial number of the wishes—especially in his region.

"I've really been thinking about this a lot since you reached out," he told me. "The effect that wishes, sports or otherwise, have is amazing—they have phenomenally changed the way the kids approach treatment. It's almost inevitable that the child I took care of before and after the wish changes 180 degrees. Now, they've just started to come out with quantitative studies showing the tangible medical benefits, and there is starting to be real evidence that the number of doctors' visits, treatments, and hospital visits all decrease after a wish," said Dr. Scothorn. He closely follows the latest studies in this area and told me that some not-yet-published research was bearing out the proof of the benefits of wish fulfillment and showing a significant reduction in post-wish medical needs.

The most recently completed such study was published by Israeli researchers in the journal *Quality of Life Research*. A pool of children with cancer, ages five to twelve, were split into two groups. All were told they would receive a wish at some point, but half were told their wish would be granted within six months; the other half were told that they would be on a waiting list. Using questions, observations, and indices to quantify hope, positive emotions, anxiety, and health-related quality of life, the researchers found that the group who expected their wishes sooner had significantly better emotional health. They showed a decrease in their perception of their physical limitations, and researchers theorized that "It is possible that wishing enabled these children to dream about that which seemed unobtainable, out of reach, and thus created an experience of achieving the impossible."

To illustrate this effect, Dr. Scothorn gave me an example of a teenager he was treating for leukemia. "It seemed like after every chemo session he ended up back in the hospital, vomiting, side effects, it took every ounce of his effort." But then his wish, to attend the regionally all-important Duke–North Carolina college basketball game, came true. "After his wish, he immediately didn't need as much medical support. We weren't getting calls in the middle of the night that he was vomiting or lethargic. Instead he got excited about going back to school and started taking more participation in his own wellness." Today he's playing high school basketball himself. "Happiness and individual-will both have a real effect on health outcomes," said Dr. Scothorn. And we already know that their passion for sports makes people happy.

The University of Iowa Stead Family Children's Hospital knows this, too. They recently capitalized on it in an effort to help patients. When the hospital built a new addition, architects designed the twelfth floor as a wraparound observation deck with expansive views of the school's Kinnick Stadium below. The floor has a sports stadium theme, including the Press Box Café with giant flat screens on the walls, where administrators set up a college football "tailgate" on Saturdays in the fall. Almost immediately, the kids, many of whom are there for very long periods of time, started enthusiastically watching Hawkeye games, often with their parents. But it was the Iowa Wave that really upped the ante.

It started when Iowa football fan Krista Young posted a note on the Hawkeye Heaven Facebook page: "I think with the new U of I hospital addition open, Kinnick should hold a 'wave to the kids' minute during every game. Can you imagine how neat it would be to have all those fans, players & coaching staff looking up at you sending a little extra inspiration?"

★ ★ ★ ★ ★ ★ ★ ★ ★ ★ ★ ★

On video, it's a simple yet stunning display of collective kindness. If you've seen the Iowa Wave, you've probably wiped back tears. It's an acknowledgement from those Iowa fans—and now, from the visiting teams and so many others: We're pulling for you. Keep going. Fight! [I]t's a message those kids and their moms need to hear. Or to see . . . It's almost overwhelming.
—*USA Today* sports columnist George Schroeder

★ ★ ★ ★ ★ ★ ★ ★ ★ ★ ★ ★

The idea immediately went viral and when the Hawkeyes opened their season at home on September 2, 2017, between the first and second quarters the crowd of 68,000 rose in unison, turned as one, and waved—and waved and waved—at the children above them. It has happened at every game since.

Six-year-old Will Kohn had been in the hospital for 295 days when he and his parents watched the Iowa Wave for the second time, and while he was surprised the first time, the wily veteran waved back confidently. "A whole stadium turning and waving . . . it's huge," said Will's mom, Meghan.

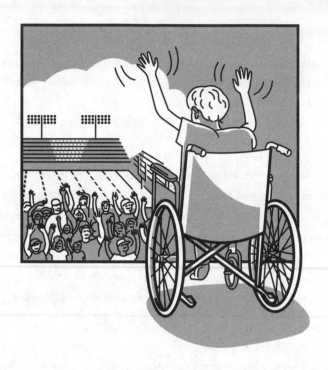

"The kids just forget about their hospital life for just a few moments." Will's dad added, "I don't think you understand it until you see it in your kid's eyes . . . you watch your child want to stay just for that." Gwen Senio, the hospital's director of child life, told *USA Today*, "It really does promote healing. And hope. It gives them hope. It gives them connection."

There's a common misconception about the Make-A-Wish Foundation—I had it myself—that it is only for the terminally ill. While that is unfortunately the case all too often, many alums survive their life-threatening illness, and the ones I spoke to who did just that all looked back at their wish fulfillment as a life-changing experience. Buddy O'Donnell spent four months in the intensive care unit and had 80 percent of his small intestine removed. He could no longer eat solid food, wore a urinary bag, and had to be fed liquid nutrients through a mediport. He was seventeen years old and his weight had dropped below one hundred pounds when the Make-A-Wish volunteers came to see him. Buddy was a lifelong sports fan who grew up watching Yankees games with his baseball-loving parents.

"I selected the baseball All-Star Game because my whole family could do it together, and it combined my two biggest passions, which still are, to this day, sports and travel," Buddy told me. "It was a life-changing trip. Doctors had told me I could never participate in sports again, but I got to see the other side of sports firsthand. Every person we met, I was like 'What do they do? That's a job in sports!' and I realized I could still participate."

Buddy did research and enrolled at the University of South Carolina for its sports entertainment management program, also got a business degree, and went on to work in high-level sales positions in the NBA, MLB, and NFL, including for the Jets, Giants, Diamondbacks, Nets, and his dream since childhood, the New York Yankees. But Buddy also found courage and inspiration and against medical advice took himself off the diet he had been told he could never change and retrained his body. Today he can eat normally again. Between job changes he has taken several unusually long trips, a few months or more, all over the world, and has skydived over Australia's Great Barrier Reef and motorbiked through Vietnam. When I spoke to him by phone, he was in Bali.

For many years Buddy did not like to talk about his Make-A-Wish experience because of all the questions it brought up, and he wouldn't take his shirt off at the beach because his torso is so heavily scarred. But when he was working for the Yankees, he realized he was finally in a position to give something back, and contacted the organization. He ended up leaving sports and working full time for the national Make-A-Wish headquarters for five years, then moving to the New Jersey chapter. In his time there, he served as a "wish escort" for kids, usually to the see the New York Giants football team, at least ten times. "I can tell you from my own personal experience, that All-Star wish has affected everything I've done the rest of my life. I've completely rebounded from where I was as a kid. I'm active, I can eat regularly; it was a game-changing experience. I went from being ashamed in my twenties to being a proud survivor. I owe it all to Make-A-Wish. But now, as a wish escort, I've seen it from the other side—over the course of a weekend you just see the change, their eyes light up."

Dr. Scothorn said, "The single most impactful sports wish I can remember involved a child who didn't survive. I was in Texas at the time and he was a huge UT fan, and that year they were playing USC in the Rose Bowl. We had a donor lined up with tickets, a plane, everything, but two days before the game, he took a turn for the worse and couldn't go. So we turned the hospital auditorium into a stadium, put the game on a TV the size of a movie theater screen, and invited all his family and friends and tried to make it just like being at the game. You could just see that there was nothing he wanted to do more than experience that game any way he could."

"A month or so later his parents came to see me at the clinic. He had been given a Rose Bowl logo hat with the teams and year on it, and they gave it to me, they wanted me to have it." Dr. Scothorn's voice started cracking as he finished the story. "It's right here on my desk in front of me, and every time I look at it . . ."

BUILDING A BETTER SPORTS FAN

*O*nce we got on the topic of physical health, I had Dr. Kristie's undivided attention. This allowed me to circle back around to her original preconception of the sports fan as slothful couch potato. So I related one of the more unexpected results, at least to me: that being a sports fan is as good for the body as for the soul. While the mental health benefits have been amply demonstrated for decades in hundreds of studies worldwide, the proposition that being a sports fan is also good for your physical health is a murkier one. Yet there is too much evidence to dismiss it—even if, admittedly, some of that evidence sounds pretty far-fetched.

For starters, a growing body of literature shows a direct connection between watching sports as a spectator and becoming a participant via fandom. Many of us play sports or do exercise because we were pushed in that direction by parents or peers, signed up for Little League, swim club, or

Tae Kwon Do lessons, or were taught to ski, as Dr. Kristie and I were doing on this fine Wyoming winter's day. But in other cases, simply being a fan, though generally thought of as a passive activity, drives us to get up and become an active participant.

I asked psychologist Leeja Carter whether spectator sports were a viable pathway toward more physical activity by its fans? Dr. Carter is a sports psychology practitioner and women's health advocate. She answered:

> Absolutely. I think that's one of the benefits of sport, one of the beauties of sport. I was just thinking about just this very topic, and one of the things about sports is that we admire athletes as role models and one of the things that makes them role models is that they have had similar life experiences to us as it relates to physical activity. Let's take Michael Phelps for example. At the age of seven he was introduced to water. So, for a kid seeing that, his introduction to physical activity and his decision to stay with that sport and become this competitive icon, that is something that is relatable to kids and to parents everywhere. By virtue of that we see the possibility of what athletics can do for us. Absolutely I think that kids and adults find inspiration in athletes,

looking at their bodies and their health, and while we might not want to become that high-level athlete, we see the potential of what our bodies can do by watching athletes.

In 2012 a group of researchers from the University of North Carolina and Duke University's Center for Cognitive Neuroscience and Departments of Psychiatry and Psychology & Neuroscience tried to determine the identity of the "typical" sports spectator, and found they enjoyed both psychological and physical advantages: "Our results indicate that individuals who report higher levels of sports spectating tend to have higher levels of extraversion, and in particular excitement seeking and gregariousness. These individuals also engage more in complementary pastime activities, including participating in sports and exercise activities . . ." It remains unclear whether being fans made them more active, or whether more active people choose to be sports fans, but there is plenty of evidence suggesting that at least some of it is due to the former.

The highest profile example of fandom leading to exercise is the Olympics, which like clockwork, now come every two years. These global spectacles typically expose huge audiences to an array of very varied athletic pursuits, many of which viewers have never tried, inspiring curiosity.

★ ★ ★ ★ ★ ★ ★ ★ ★ ★ ★ ★

I had got into the Olympic spirit and felt it was time to get myself fit, and quit smoking. To start with I joined a gym.
—Alex Griffin, British college student,
after watching the 2012 London Olympic Games

★ ★ ★ ★ ★ ★ ★ ★ ★ ★ ★ ★

In one study, the Sporting Goods Manufacturers Association, the largest global trade group for manufacturers and retailers in the sports products industry, tracked participation rates for sports included in the 2008 Beijing Summer Olympics. The year following the Games saw double-digit growth in triathlon participation, arguably the single most fitness-oriented recreational sport of all, as well as jumps of 5 to 7 percent each in running, cycling, and beach volleyball. All of these are sports that have very little mainstream television coverage outside of the Olympic Games, strongly suggesting that it was the very act of watching them that caused the spikes in participation— or as I see it, more people exercised because they had watched sports on TV. According to research by the International Academy of Sports Science and Technology, the last games held in this country, the 2002 Salt Lake Winter Olympics, "had a positive impact on the physical activity levels country-wide."

The most recent example was the historic success of the US Women's Cross-Country Ski Team at the 2018 Winter Games in South Korea winning the nation's first-ever gold medal in a pastime long dominated by Scandinavian countries. This immediately caused newcomers to try the sport, according to Marie-Ange Anderson, activities director at Colorado's Devil's Thumb Ranch, ranked the best Nordic resort ski center in the nation, and who saw the effect firsthand. Within weeks of the Games, she told me, newcomers were showing up for rentals and lessons to give Nordic skiing a try and telling her it was because of watching the Olympics.

Every Olympic Games debuts a few new sports, and fans of surfing and rock climbing were eagerly anticipating the 2020 Tokyo Games, where both would be showcased on the global Olympic stage for the first time. Like Nordic skiing, beach volleyball, or triathlons, these get very little traditional prime time coverage, yet they seem to lend themselves to the model of inspiring viewers to give them a try. Surfing is a dynamic, exciting, and beautiful undertaking, and, like skiing, it is showcased in the Games at the highest level but is also very welcoming to beginners, and accessible at coastlines all over the globe. The form of climbing to be judged in Tokyo, an indoor wall style, is even more receptive to curious fans, as it can be safely tried in gyms anywhere, including in the world's largest cities. If the postponed Tokyo Games cannot be held in 2021 (dependent on the state of the coronavirus pandemic), surfing and climbing will not get their chance at a high-profile moment until Paris 2024.

There is also a theory in the sports industry that, in addition to the novel sports, witnessing the athletes themselves, chiseled role models for fitness and athletic performance, inspires viewers to get in shape even without taking up new sports. After Beijing, researchers found sizable participation jumps in sixteen very different fitness pursuits, most of them gym-based, from using elliptical trainers and weights to joining classes such as yoga and cardio kickboxing.

★ ★ ★ ★ ★ ★ ★ ★ ★ ★ ★ ★

While some people may not be motivated to play a particular sport because of watching the Olympic Games, many people are encouraged to start exercising and getting in better physical shape because of the Olympic Games . . . In some cases, we see a straight line from Olympic coverage and increased sports participation . . . The research clearly supports that analysis.
—Neil Schwartz of SGMA Research in an industry report

★ ★ ★ ★ ★ ★ ★ ★ ★ ★ ★ ★

"What's really exciting for us is that it happens both in the Winter Olympics and the Summer Olympics, so we get a really good cycle every two years," Carl Liebert, former president and CEO of 24 Hour Fitness, said, after the chain, one of America's largest national health club operators, saw a surge in new memberships in the next hundred days following the 2012 London Games. Similar Olympic-inspired surges were reported at other individual and chain gyms all around the world.

What is more debatable is whether these surges last. Just as many self-improvement-based New Year's resolutions are infamously short lived, post-Olympic studies have shown wildly different results on longer-term outcomes, depending on the country and the sports on which they have been conducted. After the 2000 Sydney Olympics, researchers found no long-term effect on the exercise habits of Australians, while Britain saw a respectable 1.3 percent increase in the numbers of citizens doing at least thirty minutes per week of moderately active exercise after the 2012 London Games (though this is an extremely low bar, below World Health Organization minimal recommendations). The 1992 Barcelona Games seemingly induced huge participation gains in the Spanish public afterward, but many researchers now think these numbers are flawed. To further confuse things, two recent studies in Canada seemed to come to opposite conclusions. One found that there were significant spikes in tennis and rowing participation after the 2008 Beijing Olympics, and similarly big upticks in curling and cross-country skiing after the 2006 Torino Winter Games. But another Canadian study found no increases in alpine skiing participation whatsoever after the nation hosted its own 2010 Winter Games in Vancouver.

However long they last, I would argue that any surges in fitness activity are beneficial, especially if they continue to be induced anew every twenty-four months. And it's likely they certainly last for some subset of the spectator population, even if it is small. There are several other fandom examples that may provide clearer evidence than the Olympics.

The current American obesity and inactivity problems are extremely well-documented, a costly and dangerous health crisis in this country. If sports fandom offers a direct path for creating a more active citizenry, that can only be positive. There is no clearer example than cycling, a sport I know that Dr. Kristie enjoys. So, I bring up the "Lance Armstrong Effect," by which tens of thousands of average, non-cycling Americans were converted into recreational cyclists—for exercise, pleasure, and long-distance charity events—a phenomenon accompanied by an equally dramatic spike in bike commuting in cities nationwide.

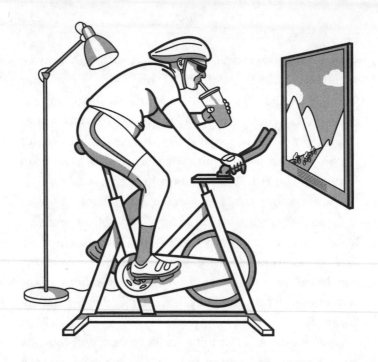

This all happened because the now-disgraced, then–American hero Lance Armstrong raised public awareness of and interest in the sport, and televised viewing of cycling in this country. In short, he created a sizable base of new sports fans, and then those fans got up off the couch and took up the sport they now paid attention to, similar to the post-Olympic surges, but even more observable—and more clearly showing longer-term staying power.

"Somewhat improbably, even as the house of cards on which Armstrong built his success collapsed amid the doping allegations, passion for the sport has not waned," wrote Steve Lipsher for the *Denver Post*. " . . . USA Cycling, the sport's national governing body, has seen the number of racer licenses climb by 45 percent [in a decade] since 2004, ranging from low-level citizen racers to elite future stars, according to spokesman Bill Kellick. 'People are still riding their bikes for all the right reasons,' he said, acknowledging that much of that increased interest is due to Armstrong. 'A sport such as cycling that isn't mainstream in the United States probably wouldn't be where it is without him and what he did.'"

Lipsher also pointed out that participation in amateur racing reversed years of decline, bike commuting and leisure riding increased, sales of bicycles skyrocketed, and an entire training empire of hundreds of specialized coaches appeared, many of them helping cyclists prepare for the vastly expanded number of charity centuries, or hundred-mile fun rides, something we can also attribute to Armstrong fandom. According to Canada's CBC News, the Lance Armstrong Effect took road bikes from a tiny fraction of the bicycle market in 2000 to nearly two-thirds of all bikes sold, a quantum leap that has mostly remained in place even since Armstrong left the sport (the currently red-hot subcategory is "gravel grinders," beefier road bikes designed to be used on both paved and unpaved surfaces). CBC reported that "the Lance Armstrong effect transformed sport and commuter cycling in general, and also played a huge role in launching the now ubiquitous charity bike-a-thon."

In turn, it is reasonable to surmise that the growth of charitable cycling events and their ability to attract non-avid cyclists likely set an example for similar booms in charity walk-a-thons, 5K and 10K "fun runs," and even gyms that have gotten into the act with indoor stationary biking and rowing machine "marathons" for charity. Every year my wife and I ride a charity cycling century in New England called the Prouty, which raises money for cancer research and treatment. Coming up on its fortieth year, in the pre-Armstrong era the Prouty attracted mainly enthusiastic cycling hobbyists. Today it draws more than four thousand annual participants and offers no fewer than sixteen different options including six road cycling lengths (twenty, thirty-five, fifty, seventy-seven, one hundred, and two hundred miles), a sixty-five-mile "gravel grinder" dirt road ride, five walking routes from 3K to 10K, rowing on the Connecticut River (five, ten, or fifteen miles), and a Virtual Prouty where participants create their own endeavor someplace else—these have come from as far away as a treadmill at the International Space Station.

While the physical health and fitness benefits associated with being a sports fan seem most pronounced when they turn sedentary citizens into more active ones, researchers have noted a couple of other ways in which being a sports fan may play a positive physical health role. I say "may," because some of this logic seems best taken with a grain of salt. According to *Prevention* magazine, "Watching live sports is a workout in itself . . . it can help you torch some calories without even trying. The average 150-pound woman burns more than 100 calories per hour attending a live sporting event. And that's just while sitting! Walking from your car to the stadium, then up eight or more flights of stairs to your seat, is another way to easily torch a few more calories, not to mention leaping from the bench when your team scores a touchdown." That all makes sense, but then again, by following this line of reasoning, so do the fitness benefits of going to a rock concert, commuting to work in a big city, or shopping at the supermarket, pushing your cart up and down the aisle, reaching for foods on higher and lower shelves, then carrying loaded bags to your car.

Using cutting-edge technology, scientists at Western Sydney University tested the hypothesis that watching sports is actually good for us in and of itself. They inserted fine needles into the nerves of participants, allowing precise recording of the electrical signals directed to blood vessels. This is considered a very sensitive and accurate measure of the body's physiological response. After obtaining baseline readings, test subjects watched video footage of a person jogging, and as a result, their breathing and heart rates accelerated—researchers concluded that they were exercising simply by watching sport. Their physical activity levels returned to normal passivity once they stopped watching the runner. According to *Medical Daily*, "Overall, the findings showed that muscle sympathetic nerve activity—the traffic of nerve impulses to the muscles—increases when people watch physical activity." And that's a good thing.

One of the researchers, Vaughan Macefield, a professor of integrative physiology, explained: "We know that the sympathetic nervous system—which supplies the heart, sweat glands, and blood vessels, as well as other tissues—increases its activity during actual exercise, and now we have shown that it increases when you are watching a moving scene [physically, not emotionally, moving] as if you were running yourself." To be fair, the doctors did not recommend watching sports as a replacement for doing sports, and were quick to note that "nothing can replace the health benefits of getting off the couch," but it could be an added plus for the sports fan.

It could also be a ridiculous conclusion, as I could find no evidence of scientists doing similar measurements on people watching horror movies or other programming you might expect to cause elevated heart rate and other similar physical responses. As much as I might want to believe that watching sports is some sort of cure-all, I'd have to see a lot more evidence—and control groups—before I swap riding my bike for the flat screen. I do, however, strongly believe that via the participation effect inspired by Lance Armstrong and other athletes, spectating can have a real positive health and fitness effect on an American population that is increasingly in need of it. In fact, I have personally experienced this—and it greatly altered my life.

"Remember when you and I used to go running when you were in medical school in Hanover?" I asked Dr. Kristie.

"Of course. With my crazy schedule it was hard to stay consistent about working out, but you pushed me to keep getting out there. Thanks again."

"Don't thank me, thank sports fandom."

In New England, where I live, the Boston Marathon is a much higher profile spectator event than any other running competition, in part because of its rich history and also because it is always held on a Massachusetts state holiday, Patriots' Day, the third Monday in April. Created to honor the inaugural Olympic Marathon of the modern era held in London in 1896—the race in which the current 26.2-mile distance was formalized after centuries of differing, random "marathon" lengths—the Boston race launched the following year, 1897. It is the oldest marathon in the country, one of six "majors" in the sport worldwide, and one of just three high-profile American sporting events that have been held continuously through both World Wars (along with the Kentucky Derby and Rose Bowl). It is New

England's most-attended sporting event, as enthusiastic spectators line the streets of the long race route, and one spring back in the early 1990s, my friend Mary watched it on television.

★ ★ ★ ★ ★ ★ ★ ★ ★ ★ ★ ★

I do imagine a great deal of that popularity and growth in cycling is seeded in people watching the Tour de France on television for the first time. If fandom opens the door to it, well that's a pretty significant thing.
—*Wall Street Journal* sports columnist and avid cyclist Jason Gay, as told to the author

★ ★ ★ ★ ★ ★ ★ ★ ★ ★ ★ ★

Like many Americans, my circle of friends all vaguely thought that we "should get more exercise," but we weren't doing anything about it. After watching the race, Mary was inspired and floated the notion that we start running, something I had never done. I figured, why not? I already owned a pair of sneakers, gym shorts, and a T-shirt, which seemed to make me fully prepared. Mary and I started with two miles—a distance that turned out to be much longer than it sounded and left me feeling like I had run the Boston Marathon. Nonetheless, we kept at it, a couple of times a week, and after a month moved up to three miles, and then four. Baby steps, as they say. The following winter, Mary suggested we run a half-marathon, which sounded like an epic distance, a real challenge, and a training goal that both motivated and terrified me.

The 13.1-mile race was the first organized running event I had ever participated in, and lining up for the start, my nerves were tingling. But much to my surprise, the race was easier than I'd anticipated, as we were swept up in the camaraderie, cheered on by roadside supporters, and refueled with water and energy drink at stands every two miles or so—something we had never had on our training runs. Instead of the relief I had anticipated upon finishing, there was excitement, accomplishment, a sense of "what's next?"

Because I had not actually watched the Boston Marathon (to be frank, I still can't imagine anything more boring than watching professionals run down city streets for over two hours), it never really registered with me before working on this book how much this one spectator event positively impacted my life. Mary was the catalyst, the one motivated by sports on TV, and had she not been, I would likely have never started running and almost certainly would not have run that first half-marathon. I would not have then run dozens more races that length over the next two decades, along with lots of 10Ks; the Philadelphia, Chicago, and Honolulu marathons; a couple of 50K (31-plus miles) trail runs; and lengthy team relays. I would not have woken up early, five days each week for years, to join a daily group for six to eight miles. I certainly would never have reached the point where that once seemingly unattainable half–marathon felt like rolling out of bed, requiring no special preparation.

I never would have bought an often-used treadmill for my home, continued running in hotel gyms around the world while on the road, or started weekly workouts with my local track club. My running experience fueled more earnest pursuit of my current passion—road cycling—along with cross-country skiing, hiking, and my lifelong interest in fitness in general. While my participation in road cycling predated the Lance Armstrong Effect, many of my friends were inspired by Armstrong, giving me a larger community of comrades on wheels, more group rides for motivation, and many more events to participate in. I know I have lived a much healthier and more fulfilling life over the past quarter century, thanks to sports on TV.

I'm hardly the only one.

According to Dr. Wann, "A number of empirical investigations have found that sports fans are as particularly likely to participate in sports as athletes . . ." Which is to say, more than the average non-fan, non-athlete. His own research shows that college-age sports fans are not only more likely to participate in athletics than non-fans, but they are also better students and devote more energy to study and involvement in the collegiate setting. Wann has also found additional health benefits besides increased participation in fitness activities. As he told me, "What fandom brings to us physically is vitality, vigor, a boost of energy, and a sense of being alive." His studies have variously found that sports fans enjoy "higher levels of vigor" and "less fatigue." But the biggie for our society is transforming fans into participants, and when I described my marathon experience, he nodded in agreement, "The fact that you are a fan makes it more likely that you are also a participant. We've seen that in the studies."

There are few better examples of the motivation effect getting spectators onto the field than the US Women's Soccer Team winning it all at the 1999 World Cup—a scenario that is now replaying itself following the highly publicized success of the team's march to another World Cup Championship in 2019. Soccer is still a relatively small spectator sport in the US, especially compared to the "big four" (football, basketball, baseball, and hockey), but in 1999 it was much less popular than it is today. Nonetheless, the team and its star players became overnight sensations, and according to sports historian Richard O. Davies, "The march of the American women to the title was followed closely by the American people . . . 79,000 wildly enthusiastic fans turned out at the Meadowlands near New York City for the Americans' trouncing of Denmark in the opening round: observers noticed that the lines of young girls at the ice cream stands were much longer than those of adults at beer concessions. Fans came with their faces painted red, white, and blue, carrying homemade banners and waving American flags. Women's sports in America had come of age."

Ninety-two thousand fans—including President Clinton—were in attendance for the final win against China in Pasadena, CA, and according to Davies, superstar Mia Hamm and her teammates "helped lure hundreds of thousands of youngsters into youth soccer programs." Hundreds of thousands! Arguing in support of the participation effect on women and girls playing soccer via the publicity of the World Cup, University of Michigan professor and sports culture expert Andrei Markovits wrote, "Very few, if any, American and European women played this game in the late 1960s and early 1970s, but millions do today—case closed!" It was a watershed moment for the fan-to-participant transformation, and to honor the occasion, a special Mia Hamm–edition Soccer Barbie Doll was released—it could say "I can kick and throw like Mia Hamm"—with some of the proceeds going to Hamm's nonprofit foundation. "When I was little, Barbie rode around in a red Corvette and lived in a mansion. I sure didn't relate to that," said Hamm. "Soccer Barbie is a lot more realistic."

This spectator-to-participant transformation has played out in various ways again and again throughout the history of sports. Twenty-year-old Francis Ouimet, a former caddie, shocked the world by defeating golf's royalty, Harry Vardon (inventor of the now-standard way of holding the club, the Vardon grip) to win the 1913 US Open in a real-life Cinderella story, as recounted in the classic book, *The Greatest Game Ever Played*. Golf was a notoriously elitist game and Ouimet, whose father was a gardener and handyman, had upended the sport. Golf boomed and newbies flocked to the course. "Ouimet's stunning victory swept golf onto the front pages of American newspapers. A working-class American had . . . awakened the American people to the exciting possibilities of golf. Middle-class American men and women began to take up the game in the 1920s as public courses opened in most cities. By 1925, an estimated 2.5 million Americans played the game," wrote Davies.

This was just the first leg of what would become the Ouimet Hagen Jones triumvirate, which forever established golf as a participant sport in this country. Another homegrown middle-class hero, Walter Hagen, won the US Open the year after Ouimet, quickly amassed more Major titles, became the first American to cross the Atlantic and win the British Open (he would do it three times), and won four consecutive PGA Championships—a record unlikely to ever be broken. Then Bobby Jones appeared on the scene, and as the game's last great amateur (he famously never turned pro), the lawyer who moonlighted as a golfer won thirteen Majors, including the Grand Slam (all four in the same year)—before abruptly retiring at age twenty-eight. When Jones arrived on the radar of sports fans in the early twenties there were fewer than five hundred courses in the country, mostly private, but by the end of the decade there were around six thousand, nearly five thousand of them public. While golf may not be viewed as the most physically intense sport, an eighteen-hole round covers an average of around five miles, and at the time of Ouimet, Hagen, and Jones, before the mechanized golf cart, all players walked the course. Many still do.

Without its relatable and inspiring role models, golf might have remained a pure spectator sport of elite specialist professionals, like equestrian jumping or sailing regattas, rather than a widespread, traditional recreation pursuit. (While golf has maintained a reputation of elitism thanks to its often very exclusive and expensive private clubs and high-profile public courses seen on television such as Pebble Beach, which typically cost over $600 to play, the reality is different. Golfers are an extremely diverse population in socio-economic terms; three quarters of the courses in the United States are very much public and the median peak-season weekend greens fees in 2019 were just $36, with lower rates available on weekdays, at off hours, and through replay or multi-round deals and other specials.)

TWENTY-FIRST CENTURY SPORTS FANS: *AMERICAN NINJA WARRIOR*

"*D*o you watch *American Ninja Warrior*?" I asked Dr. Kristie.

"No. I've heard of it, but I don't know anything about it. Do you?"

"Yes, I've become obsessed with it. There is no other sport I set my DVR to record every episode of. I highly recommend it."

In addition to the jaw-dropping displays of athleticism, what really fascinates me about the show is how it has become a shining example of the fan–turned–active participant paradigm. If I were younger, fitter, and born with better coordination, I'd be tempted to give it a go myself.

ANW is not like any other sport on television, and appears to be the only full–season, non–team sport regularly broadcast in prime time on a major network, filling a void left many years ago by the end of once ultra-popular boxing coverage. In the summer of 2018, NBC, which had once successfully aired Friday Night Fights (technically titled *Gillette Cavalcade of Sports*) from Madison Square Garden for fourteen years, used *American Ninja Warrior* to take control of Monday night prime time as the top-rated network. *American Ninja Warrior* pulled in an impressive five to six million weekly viewers in its eighth season, making it one of the more popular shows on television.

For the uninitiated, *ANW* is an obstacle course race that continuously invents new, complex, sometimes bizarre, and often incredibly difficult individual obstacles, linked together into courses of increasing length. Competitors who go the furthest each week advance, first to city finals and then national finals. Because each contestant gets just one shot, the all-or-nothing format adds considerably to the drama, as even proven veterans, crowd favorites, and the world's best can—and often do—see their entire season end with a single missed step, poorly judged handhold, or mistimed aerial maneuver on signature obstacles such as the "salmon ladder," "propeller bar," or "jumping spider."

It requires unbelievable athleticism coupled with unrelenting attention, and to up the tension, many of the competitors are compulsively consumed by speed and the bragging rights of finishing a course fastest, even though it inspires reckless abandon which often leads to season-ending mistakes, and despite that fact that this has not traditionally given them any advantage (a bonus was added in the 2019 season for the two fastest in each city, though this does not affect most participants). Imagine not getting an extra point for the two-point conversion in the NFL and going for it anyway, just because it's fun to try?

If the competitors do everything right and get past the first stage of National Finals in Las Vegas, which about thirty typically do in a massive culling of the season's talent (in 2019, about six hundred competed nationwide of which eighty-six qualified for the finals and twenty-eight survived round one), they move on to two special and much harder stages, which they must complete in order to attempt a climb of the season's very last obstacle, Mount Midoriyama. The show is an officially recognized American adaptation of one created in Japan (there are now several Ninja Warrior shows worldwide and even international Ryder Cup-style US versus the World competitions), and Mount Midoriyama is a near carbon copy of the Japanese one with the same name, recreated annually alongside the neon lights of the Las Vegas Strip.

One of the more fascinating aspects about *ANW* is that other than endorsements or opening training gyms or motivational speaking or otherwise parlaying success into ancillary benefits the athletes secure on their own, no participants seem to make any money. Until 2018, the entire concept hinged on a million-dollar prize for conquering the last two near-impossible stages and Mount Midoriyama—a task so difficult that after nine full seasons, the network has only signed one check. In 2018, only two of the thirty finalists made it through stage two, and neither got halfway through the third course. Unlike every other sport on television, nearly every season ends without a clear champion, though in 2018 the show added a $100,000 prize for the season's "last ninja standing." They also added a few $10,000 performance bonuses along the way, but less than 1 percent of the competitors who make it onto television each year (many trained and exceptionally fit wannabe ninjas don't even get that far) get anything at all, and most actually spend money to compete.

As a spectator, to me the thrill comes in several ways, and the drama of whether they will finish the course or not, never a given at any level, keeps me glued to each participant's run. But ultimately, it's the nonstop barrage of stupefying acts of physical strength and athletic ability that wow even the uninformed. There are moments like that watching football, when a receiver makes an unbelievable one-handed diving catch with a defender draped all over him, or a possessed linebacker throws aside offensive linemen like scraps of paper for a shockingly efficient and relentless sack, but these come only occasionally, and this is true in most sports. *American Ninja Warrior,* on the other hand, is a nonstop highlight reel of athletic prowess, constantly redefining the very notion of what is physically possible. It's also very relatable in its difficulty—I can imagine catching a pass or making a three-pointer, but I cannot imagine moving through a long procession of doorknobs hanging from the ceiling overhead using only my fingers because I know how hard that is. I'm on the edge of my seat the entire show, and I know my mirror neurons are firing on all cylinders.

While I can definitively say you will never see me swinging from rope to rope or trying to run up the "Mega-Wall," lots of other people are doing exactly these things in one of the most demonstrable examples of sports spilling over from the flat screen into our personal lives. Because it is an entirely new kind of sport, the show's popularity has created an entirely new kind of gym, the "ninja training gym," and these have exploded in popularity across the country. I think it's safe to assume that like most people who take boxing classes or practice karate or run without professional or Olympic aspirations, the majority of the people training at these gyms understand that they will never be on the show. Thus, it is hard to argue that the thousands of people now working out intensely have been motivated by anything else but by being fans of a spectator sport—fandom that translates directly into their well-being. Of course, some of them may have an inner need for fitness or exercise they would have fulfilled some other way, but during the backstories in almost every episode we meet parents who describe how their kids had no interests or outlets until *ANW* came along and inspired them. Sometimes these adults tell the same stories about themselves, after a lifetime of not finding another fitness activity.

The impact is concretely observable, because when the show debuted eleven years ago, there were exactly zero ninja gyms in this country. By mid-2018 there were more than two hundred, spread across at least forty-three states. Less than a year later, as of July 2019, that number had increased by more than 50 percent, with the *Ninja Guide* website listing more than 330 gyms, located in every state except Delaware, West Virginia, and Mississippi—and that list is almost surely incomplete. "People are looking for some way to exercise that keeps them motivated and keeps their attention, and these gyms are that," said Anthony Storm, executive producer for the show, adding, "The growth of the ninja-warrior gym has been exponential."

Steve Kimpton, instructor and founder of a ninja gym called Arizona on the Rocks, believes they are proliferating because the show has gone mainstream. "This form of unique training is becoming more and more popular every season as more fans tune in." One popular contestant even launched a business designing and installing ninja obstacle courses in people's backyards.

"Inspired by the television series *American Ninja Warrior*, where contestants tackle challenging obstacles, kids and adults alike are climbing, jumping, and swinging their way into obstacle-style fitness," wrote the *Baltimore Sun*, which found that its region now had at least three dedicated ninja gyms offering courses for all ages. Heather Crowe, clinical associate professor of kinesiology at Towson University, sees several benefits in the trend, especially as a way to get kids interested in exercising at a young age, along with the fact that these workouts can be done almost anywhere, cheaply, and with minimal equipment, including playgrounds, backyards, or the great outdoors. She found other good things about the ninja training fitness craze: because this kind of training lends itself to participation by the whole family, it's a new twist on the multigenerational bonding that has long been found in spectator sports, but with more of a fitness upside.

We aspire to become what we see on the screen . . .
Instead of simply being a show on a screen,
American Ninja Warrior has become a catalyst
that leads people to try something new.
**—Case Lawrence, CEO of indoor trampoline
and extreme sports park chain CircusTrix**

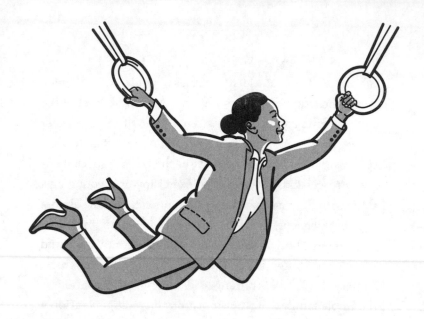

Wall Street Journal sportswriter Jason Gay penned a column called "Is 'American Ninja Warrior' the Future of Sports?" and tried to explain its popularity. "Ninjas come from every walk of life: There are ex-jocks, students, veterans, cops, lawyers, artists, EMTs. There have been autistic ninjas and legally blind ninjas . . . *Ninja Warrior* believes that despite all of its athleticism, what may matter most is accessibility. The people on the show appear to be like people you know. They fail. They fail again. Maybe one day they succeed, maybe they don't. But they try . . ." Right now, thousands of Americans, from children to seniors, are trying, and it is making them healthier. Which is a good thing.

BAD FANS OR BAD ROLE MODELS?

*A*fter another exhilarating run, Dr. Kristie and I were again on the chairlift and I returned to our conversation about the Lance Armstrong Effect. "The surge in cycling around Lance Armstrong's popular celebrity also created a surge of charity rides in communities all across the country. For each of these hundreds of events held each year, there are many people who wouldn't otherwise ride at all who commit to doing fifty, seventy-five, or a hundred miles several months in advance. To do that, they have to train. So while these may just be one- or two-day events, in preparation they are getting out there on weekends or after work for months, or going to the gym and taking spin classes. That all starts with fandom, and it's got to be good for society, right?"

Dr. Kristie nodded approvingly. Then the other shoe dropped. "But what about the drugs and cheating?" she countered, referring to Armstrong. "He's hardly a good role model."

She had me there, and I agreed wholeheartedly. As much as I've come to love the effects of spectator sports on its fans and society as whole, this is the biggest exception, the worst thing about our passion for "the game." The bad-apple athlete—and the fans who condone such behavior in the name of hero worship—are all too real. Fortunately, though, they remain exceptions, not the rule.

Lance Armstrong was hardly the first, or last, professional competitor disgraced by drugs, performance enhancing or recreational. Many of his peers have demonstrated even worse behavior, including murder, assault, domestic violence, other criminal acts of assorted kinds, hateful speech, and so on and so on. This ethically and criminally bad behavior by athletes is the first part of the worst aspect of spectator sports. The second part is on the fans: one athlete behaving badly is one person, but the spectators who accept that behavior are legion.

When athletes fail us, we are often culpable. This is the biggest downside I have seen of fandom, how our admiration for physical talent or the boost even a badly flawed individual can give "our" team often overrides common decency. There have certainly been worse examples than Michael Vick, but as a lifelong, avid dog lover, he is my personal example of loathing. A highly talented star NFL quarterback, Vick was warmly welcomed back by many fans after serving jail time for sadistically fighting dogs to the death against one another, in a horribly cruel, elaborate, systematic, and long-running criminal enterprise uncovered by law enforcement in 2007. It was not an accident or a case of bad judgment or a one-time thing; it was a lifestyle. And though his fans have tried, there is simply no way to excuse it. Yet while I blame Vick for a lot of things, wanting to come back and make millions more in the NFL is not one of them. I blame the team's management and ownership for letting him return despite what he had done, making the Philadelphia Eagles organization de facto endorsers of animal cruelty.

The Eagles have a rich history, with lots of all-time great players and coaches, including the improbable story of Vince Papale, a thirty-year-old local bartender who battled his way into the NFL through sheer grit and determination. Papale was the inspiration for the Mark Wahlberg film *Invincible*. Philly fans are among the most passionate of all sports fans—which is really saying something—and I was thrilled when they enthusiastically lined up for almost the entire route of the city's marathon and gave me and thirty thousand other runners great support. But to me, the team's current owner and executives squandered the eighty-seven-year-old franchise's history.

In the past decade, several dozen athletes in the three biggest professional sports leagues (NBA, NFL, MLB) have faced serious allegations of sexual assault or domestic violence, yet only a small handful were punished in any way at all by their respective league or team. This terrible conduct is also made possible by fan complacency. If fans voted with their wallets not to accept such behavior, profit-driven owners would be much more eager and willing to take action. This is a fair assumption, because we've just seen it happen—the NFL's current concussion crisis played out exactly along these lines.

While complaints and lawsuits from former players, as well as mounting scientific evidence, initially did little to inspire league action, the fast-growing—and admittedly belated—response by a growing number of fans to turn away from the sport altogether had an impact and sent the league scurrying into rule changes to better protect players and reduce the violent impacts and long-term danger. The NFL enacted a significant new rule limiting helmet-to-helmet contact before the 2018 season. In years before and since, sports writers have penned opinion columns about why they can no longer watch football, and the *Atlantic* considered whether simply watching the game is ethical. As publicity surrounding concussion problems soared, especially after the league's billion-dollar 2016 lawsuit settlement, and 2015 Will Smith movie *Concussion*, ratings dropped significantly the following season. While this could have had a number of other causes, most news outlets, from NBC to *Fortune*, as well as the Gallup Poll, attributed concussions as a major factor.

In the first full regular season after the new NFL helmet rule was in place, the results appeared dramatic—the number of concussions throughout the regular season dropped by nearly a third from the previous year, a substantial reduction, while clearly the athletes on the field did not get slower, smaller, or weaker.

There is more to do, of course. Concussions remain a very real problem for sports, not just football, but the good news is that this example shows fans can affect positive change, but they need to do this more, and be less accepting of criminal or unacceptable behavior. The bad news is that when fans turn a blind eye to athlete transgressions, even very serious ones, they are changing their own internal moral compasses and becoming part of the problem.

When New England Patriots star quarterback Tom Brady was caught playing with intentionally underinflated footballs in what became known as the "Deflategate" scandal, he received a four-game suspension. In the long term, this was no big deal, and the relatively minor punishment probably fit the relatively minor offense, and should have been over, done, and swept into the dustbin of history in a month. But Pats fans rallied to his support, despite the fact that his team had been very publicly caught cheating not long before (a video signal-stealing scheme), under the same management, coach, and owner, and that the conclusion of his guilt by the NFL's investigation was backed by the United States Court of Appeals. But many Patriots fans didn't care about guilt, or that he had broken the rules—they just wanted him on the field, winning. So, they began donning "Free Brady" T-shirts, a sentiment usually reserved for Nelson Mandela–like figures under unjust imprisonment. The humor was lost on me, because while Brady was getting paid millions to not take hits for a few weeks, his supporters saw that as justification to mock the terrible reality of real victims of injustice wrongly jailed by totalitarian regimes around the world. The reason for this unfortunate choice of messaging was the simple fact that to some fans, what good he could do for their favorite team outweighed what bad he had been doing when he was caught cheating.

My research assistant, sports fan Kasey Storey—it was her mother, Kelly, who ran on the treadmill to a cardboard John Elway and leveraged her lifelong passion for the Denver Broncos to overcome bone cancer—is bright and intro-spective, so I asked her if she thought her fandom had ever caused her to overlook bad athlete behavior. Without hes-itation, she answered yes: "In terms of my moral compass being altered by my sports fandom, the biggest example I can think of is indeed Lance Armstrong. We love the Tour de France at my house, and we were all avid supporters of Lance Armstrong. My whole family wore Livestrong bracelets [the once very popular yellow rubber bracelets supporting Armstrong's cancer charity Livestrong, with which he is no longer associated], especially since we had a personal experience with cancer in the family. When all of his cheating was unearthed, I remember writing a post about still wearing my yellow bracelet and supporting Lance no matter what . . . I certainly did not feel the same way about Floyd Landis when he was caught." (Armstrong's onetime teammate Landis was the next American racer to have a Tour de France championship voided for cheating with performance enhancing drugs, leaving three-time winner Greg LeMond as the only US cyclist to win the sport's biggest event.)

"No matter what" is the part that worries me most about Kasey and many other fans, especially given that Armstrong was not simply caught cheating, but also of running a complex and dedicated years-long systematic cover-up scheme. He eventually had to forfeit every important win in his career and was (and is) the subject of many lawsuits. His fraud and elaborate subsequent attempts to hide it was a well-planned campaign that included blatant lies, intimidation, and ruining other racers' careers. He put his entire sport under a cloud that still obscures it today. While he has admitted his wrongs, Armstrong has remained vehemently unrepentant and combative. Yet plenty of fans like Kasey knowingly turned a blind eye to his serial cheating and lying. Why?

When fans become so enthralled of players that in their eyes the athletes can do no wrong, they are able to rationalize excusing the inexcusable—"no matter what." One of the best-known examples is that of star Baltimore Ravens running back Ray Rice, who was arrested after getting into a fight with his fiancée in an Atlantic City casino. Despite video that appeared to show Rice dragging his limp girlfriend from an elevator, his team and coaches immediately defended him, with Ravens owner Steve Bisciotti assuring fans that Rice would "definitely be back" and absurdly adding, "He's just been lauded as the nicest, hardest working, greatest guy on the team and in the community. So we have to support him."

NFL Commissioner Roger Goodell handed down a two-game suspension, hardly sending a message to fans or players that this kind of behavior was to be frowned upon (Tom Brady's later suspension for using underinflated balls was twice as long). Goodell then apparently realized, amid the outcry, the inadequacy of the Rice penalty and publicly announced that, "I take responsibility both for the decision and for ensuring that our actions in the future properly reflect our values. I didn't get it right. Simply put, we have to do better. And we will." He released a new league-wide domestic violence policy with a six-game suspension without pay for the first offense, and lifetime ban for second. Shortly thereafter, video went public of Rice punching his fiancée in the face earlier in the casino elevator incident. This time the Ravens released him, Bisciotti apologized for his earlier statements, and the NFL upgraded the suspension to indefinite (Rice appealed the suspension and an arbitrator sided with him, reversing it, but he never signed with another team and has since left the game). The moral of this story seems to be that you have to be caught red-handed doing something really egregious to lose the support of some fans (and team management) and in this case, beating your girlfriend unconscious is not bad enough unless someone films the brutal act.

I have a longtime friend who is a lawyer, a mother, and a dyed-in-the-wool Pittsburgh Steelers fan. While she voluntarily answered my questions without hesitation and knew her answers would be published, I prefer she remains anonymous. I asked her how she reconciled her fandom and her own life choices with the sexual assault allegations against her team's star quarterback Ben Roethlisberger. (In a 2010 incident, an anonymous college student alleged that Roethlisberger raped her in a bathroom stall at a Georgia nightclub. The local prosecutor declined to press charges citing lack of evidence, but the NFL suspended the star for six games, later reduced to four.) My friend told me, "I am not unlike most fans in that I tend to give 'my' team's players the benefit of the doubt when allegations about them come to light. Specifically, in the case of the bathroom bar in Georgia fiasco, I never believed he raped her. Is that because he is the quarterback of my favorite team? Maybe. But I also question the character of women who hang out at bars and chase after professional athletes. As I recall, no charges were ever filed . . . Today, he is the married father of three and does lots of charity work. He is, by any standards, one of the 'good guys' in the NFL. He worked really hard to improve his image and I have nothing but good things to say about him now both as a leader on the field and a great role model off it."

When it comes to fan rationalizations, that one is just downright scary, and more so given her acknowledgement of how Roethlisberger's role as the star of her favorite team plays in her judgment. But it is even worse in light of what her response left unsaid. I had asked about "allegations," but she chose the one she found most defensible, and ignored another, though I am sure she knows about it. A year before the nightclub incident she referred to, Roethlisberger was accused of another sexual assault by an employee of a Lake Tahoe hotel he had stayed in. That case was settled out of court and seems harder to explain away—unless you are an avid Steelers fan apparently.

Several football fans I spoke to at the time about my issues with Michael Vick responded with some close variant of "but he's so talented," as if that would bring the dogs back from the dead. The message from folks like Steve

Bisciotti is one we see again and again when athletes trans-
gress: that we want them back regardless of what they've
done because they can perform on the field, and that athleticism and hard work in practice somehow neutralizes
real-life offenses. Fortunately, like the NFL with concussions, this seems to be changing.

As spring training for baseball's 2019 season opened,
the *Chicago Sun-Times* headline covering the city's beloved
Cubs was "Russell returns to field, braces for fan wrath
over domestic-violence suspension." The "isolated boos"
that greeted Addison Russell in his first plate appearance
since serving a forty-game suspension for domestic violence, and the fact that he was only back for a "conditional
second chance," to make the team based on performance
and contrition (he ultimately failed to do so and was per-
manently cut by the Cubs), were bad news for Russell, but
I have to view it as good news for sports fans and for society. That supporters as passionate as Cubs fans, among
the staunchest in the game, could hold one of "their own"
players to higher standards than on-field performance is
a big improvement from sports' most notorious domestic
violence story, that of Rice. If the Russell example is the
new direction—and I hope it is—then fan attitudes have
improved.

SPORTS FANS AND CIVIL RIGHTS

"*I*'m glad you share my concerns about the blindness of sports fans when it comes to issues off the field," said Dr. Kristie. "For a minute there I thought you were drinking too much fan Kool-Aid. I mean it is great for society when people are happier and people are healthier, and when communities pull together after trauma, but it's not so great when they choose sports heroes over pressing issues like drugs and violence."

"You're absolutely right, sports fandom is not a cure-all, and there are problems with it. But I'd still argue that it's far more positive than negative—and even when it comes to these social issues, that's still the case. For every Michael Vick or Lance Armstrong shocking us with disgusting behavior, there are many more athletes taking the moral high ground, advocating for change, or leading by example, and in turn, fans have responded accordingly. The same platform, public attention, and regard that fans afford athletes can make our world a much better place."

"Give me an example," Dr. Kristie asked.

"How about the civil rights movement. And the women's rights movement. And the gay rights movement?"

As Michigan professor Andrei Markovits has written, "In retrospect, the story of Jackie Robinson could rightly be seen as the inauguration of the modern civil rights movement in American society . . . a critical juncture that was to change the racial composition of America's leading sports institution, irrevocably paving the way for a major shift in American culture as whole."

To fully appreciate Jackie Robinson's impact on spectators all across America, you have to first appreciate just how hugely popular and important baseball was in 1947. America lived and breathed baseball, which was more popular than the other three big pro sports combined, truly the biggest national stage. In his day, Babe Ruth, who played until 1935, just a decade before Robinson, had his photograph reproduced more times than any other human being on the planet, ever, making him recognizable to people in parts of the world who had never seen the game. Ruth died two decades before I was born, yet he remains instantly recognizable to me, and to people much younger. The most famous baseball stars were the most famous people doing anything, and Jackie Robinson, literally overnight, became the most famous baseball player.

★ ★ ★ ★ ★ ★ ★ ★ ★ ★ ★ ★ ★

Robinson's entire baseball career was a centerpiece of
the civil rights movement . . . There can be no doubt that
before Martin Luther King Jr., before Malcolm X,
and before Nelson Mandela, Jackie Robinson was . . .
our first and unquestionably most formative
Black profile in courage.
—Whitman College professor Patrick Henry in
Jackie Robinson: Race, Sports, and the American Dream

★ ★ ★ ★ ★ ★ ★ ★ ★ ★ ★ ★ ★

"Barack Obama would never have become president
without Jackie Robinson. Jackie opened that door," claimed
Ken Burns. The winner of several Emmys, Grammys,
Academy Award nominations, and a Peabody award, among
many, many other honors, Burns is known for his detailed
multi-part historical documentaries on the Civil War, the
National Parks, and jazz, and has also covered both baseball
and, separately, Robinson, in his films. "Jackie Robinson was
the most important player in the history of Major League
Baseball. Maybe not the best, but the most important."

While many would agree with Burns on this last point,
his assertion about Obama is more questionable. Leaders
of the civil rights movement such as Martin Luther King
Jr., John Lewis, Malcom X, and many others would have

continued their fight, with or without Black professional athletes. On the other hand, Robinson's role was without a doubt the most important factor in the struggle to break the color barrier in baseball, and that helped change American history.

So I think he is at least half right, and while it may be an overreach to say Obama "would never have" become president, I absolutely have to agree that Robinson "opened that door." After all, so does Obama: while standing in the Oval Office congratulating the Chicago Cubs on their historic 2016 World Series win—on Martin Luther King Day—Obama said, "[T]here's a direct line between Jackie Robinson and me standing here . . . Sometimes it's just a matter of us being able to escape and relax from the difficulties of our day, but sometimes it also speaks to something better in us. And when you see this group of folks of different shades and different backgrounds . . . that tells us a little something about what America is and what America can be. So it's entirely appropriate that we celebrate the Cubs today here in this White House on Dr. Martin Luther King's birthday because it helps direct us in terms of what this country has been, and what it can be in the future."

Reverend King himself said of Robinson and the cause, "He was a sit-inner before sit-ins, a freedom rider before freedom rides . . . back in the days when integration wasn't fashionable, he underwent the trauma and humiliation and

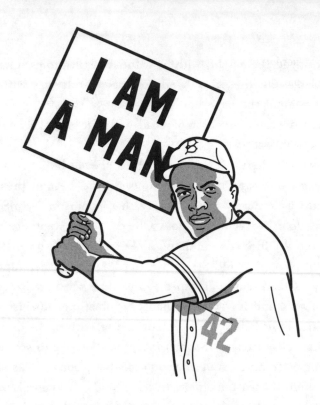

the loneliness that comes with being a pilgrim that walks in the lonesome byways toward the high road of Freedom."

The coauthors of *Sport and the Color Line* wrote, "For many Americans, Black and White alike, the desegregation of Major League Baseball represented the most important symbolic breakthrough in race relations before the 1954 Supreme Court decision in *Brown v. Board of Education*." New York sportswriter Lester Rodney echoed Ken Burns when he quoted another Black baseball pioneer, Robinson's teammate Roy Campanella, remembering that he "once said something to me like 'Without the Brooklyn Dodgers you don't have *Brown v. Board of Education* . . . we were the first ones on the trains, the first ones down South not to go around the back of the restaurant, first ones in hotels. We were like the teachers of the whole integration thing.'" Hall-of-Famer Campanella joined the team a year after Robinson, and the key to his logic was that the Dodgers were not protesting segregation, they were practicing integration, and showing fans all over the country that it could work. They were actually doing, it, living it, leading by example—and they had the platforms to make an impact.

★ ★ ★ ★ ★ ★ ★ ★ ★ ★ ★ ★

Sometimes it's not enough just to change laws. You've got to change hearts. And sports has a way sometimes of changing hearts in a way that politics or business doesn't.
—President Barack Obama

★ ★ ★ ★ ★ ★ ★ ★ ★ ★ ★ ★

Robinson, Campanella, and many athletes helped increase tolerance and decrease discrimination against Blacks, Italians, Jews, women, Muslims, the LBGTQ+ community, and various groups by changing hearts and minds.

These include Jesse Owens and Hank Greenberg, Joe Louis and Joe DiMaggio, Billy Jean King, and Muhammad Ali. Campanella's word "teachers" was an excellent choice, and this was part of what I tried to convey to Dr. Kristie: These stars did not transform the game, which was still baseball or football or basketball or boxing, they transformed the fans, who were often willing to go where their teams took them.

Psychologists who study sports fans have found that sports team allegiance is deeply ingrained and one of the most important aspects in many of our lives. Consider this: a 2017 study in the United Kingdom found that people are more than twice as likely and willing to change religions as to switch allegiance from their favorite team to another. Now think how rarely you hear of anyone you know converting to another religion.

★ ★ ★ ★ ★ ★ ★ ★ ★ ★ ★ ★

I put the obvious question to Cole. How can he risk missing a life-saving heart transplant for a football game?
"It's what I always say," he tells me. "If I can't go to Alabama football games, what's the point in living?"
—Warren St. John, *Rammer Jammer Yellow Hammer*

★ ★ ★ ★ ★ ★ ★ ★ ★ ★ ★ ★

Team allegiance often merges with a fan's identity. As a result, if a team makes changes that conflict with beliefs a fan holds, the fans are forced to confront a decision about whether to stick with their team. Those contradictory beliefs have to be extremely powerful to cause them to reject their team.

So in the spring of 1947, in a country in which segregation of everything from public restrooms to transportation to hotels and restaurants to schools was the legal and the cultural norm, if you were a Dodgers fan, and you had prejudices—as many fans did—you were suddenly faced with a big dilemma. On April 15, at Ebbets Field in Brooklyn, when for the first time in history a Black man stepped onto the diamond at a Major League Baseball game in uniform— the beloved uniform of your Dodgers—your choice was to remain a bigot and surrender your fandom, or change your heart and keep your team. This is an oversimplification.

Choosing the latter strategy, becoming more accepting of Blacks, as most Dodgers fans did, was in many cases subliminal or subconscious, and as Dr. Leeja Carter, the head of the Diversity & Inclusion Council for the Association for Applied Sport Psychology told me, "more accepting" is not the same as accepting. "While someone's racism might not be overt, it could still be covert and more subtle. With the Jackie Robinson example, individuals who had a more hostile and open form of racism might have transitioned to a more subtle form in order to remain within that sports community they felt so strongly about. I don't think sports can make someone not a racist, but they might say, I love my team so much and I recognize that the culture within it is changing and I am going to change with it and go a little more covert with my '-isms.' I do think that sports has the power to bring people's awareness of civil right issues, and to our responsibilities as humans, to become advocates and allies to other people. It's not just racism, it is all '-isms.'"

To whatever degree the changes in fan attitude were conscious or not, sweeping or subtle, overt or covert, they were nonetheless vitally important. In *The Boys of Summer*, Roger Kahn observed, "By applauding Robinson, a man did not feel that he was taking a stand on school integration, or on open housing . . . But . . . to disregard color for even an instant, is to step away from the old prejudices, the old hatred. That is not a path on which many double back."

"Minimal group theory" analyzes the psychological and social effects of groups. In one experiment, neuropsychology researcher Jay Van Bavel tested White subjects for racial bias, then assigned them to one of two imaginary mixed-race "teams," the Lions and Tigers. When he retested them, their levels of racial bias had decreased, simply because they now belonged, in name only, to a diverse group. Van Bavel concluded that "merely belonging to a mixed-race team triggers positive automatic associations with all the members of their own group, irrespective of race."

This same logic would apply to the mixed-race, -age, and -gender audiences found at most sporting events. "Every person has so many identities that they bring to the table," said Dr. Carter. "And they're coming to sports with that diversity to see athletes who are also very diverse, but there's a unifying thread, this love of competition and entertainment." Or as science writer Eric Simons put it, using Los Angeles Raiders football fans as an example, "In this crowd of men and women, young and old, Blacks, Whites, and Latinos (plus one gorilla), the only category that mattered was Silver and Black."

The path to tolerance and the role of spectator sports in advancing civil rights, human rights, and lessening discrimination and prejudice has been a slow one with many bumps in the road, yet in the seventy-plus years since Jackie Robinson, millions of sports fans around the globe have been transformed into more tolerant human beings.

That is no small thing.

After his death, Robinson's wife, Rachel, who had been through his side for the entire history-making episode, penned a memoir and wrote: "I believe that the singly most important aspect of Jack's presence was that it enabled White baseball fans to root for a Black man, thus encouraging more Whites to realize that all our destinies were inextricably linked."

In his first season, Robinson's Dodgers broke the attendance record in every National League city they visited except Cincinnati, and the League shattered its all-time overall attendance record by three-quarters of a million spectators, with five different teams—including the Dodgers—setting new season records. By the end of that very first season, five other Black players were signed by Major League teams, Robinson was on the cover of *Time* magazine, and he was named Rookie of the Year by the *Sporting News*—whose editor had been an outspoken critic of integration in the game. In fact, the hatred originally directed at Robinson did not come just from fans, but from many within baseball and even within the Dodgers clubhouse, including horribly cruel racism from teammates. Another original critic of baseball's "Great Experiment" was Red Barber, the White Southern-born Dodgers announcer at the time who found it distasteful that he had to convey Robinson's achievement to the public. Yet he too was won over, and years later, after what he described as "deep self-examination," he realized that, "I know if I have achieved any understanding and tolerance in my life . . . it all stems from this. I thank Jackie Robinson."

While inspiring Black Americans, Robinson simultaneously led White fans to reassess their own belief systems, and San Francisco State University history professor Jules Tygiel, author of two books on Robinson, wrote of his first season that "affection for Robinson grew so widespread that at the year's end voters in an annual public opinion poll named him the second most popular man in America. Only Bing Crosby registered more votes." Shockingly, that transformation took just one season and his popularity only continued to grow. It has never waned since: Robinson's number, 42, will never again be worn by anyone else, as it was the first and only number retired by every team— in every major American sport, not just baseball—and is the only one displayed in every big-league ballpark. More than seventy years after he first strode onto Ebbets Field, American sports fans still rank him as the single most popular athlete of all time.

★ ★ ★ ★ ★ ★ ★ ★ ★ ★ ★ ★

The lesson is if we can play sports together, what can't we do together? I think the very high visibility of spectator sports has been very important in breaking through all these glass barriers.
—Dr. Mark Emmert, NCAA president, as told to the author

★ ★ ★ ★ ★ ★ ★ ★ ★ ★ ★ ★

Robinson was the highest profile athlete to change fans' racist perceptions but he was not the only one. Another giant was boxer Joe Louis, who became the uncontested World Heavyweight Champion in 1937 and whose racially motivated nickname was the "Brown Bomber." But because his sole career loss had been to German fighter Max Schmeling, when he won the belt he stated publicly that he would not consider himself the champ until he was victorious in a rematch. To say the stakes were high is no hyperbole: after Black track-and-field superstar Jesse Owens stole the show at the 1936 Summer Olympics in Berlin by winning a record four gold medals, Adolf Hitler, his Aryan pride deeply wounded, put his propaganda spotlight on the 1938 fight. In the run-up to it, Hitler's staff issued statements claiming that no Black man could defeat Schmeling, and that the winning purse from the fight would be used to build more German tanks.

By the time of the rematch, the event had transcended boxing and taken on enormous global symbolism, representing the ultimate showdown between good and evil, freedom against tyranny, democracy versus Nazism. In Germany, Hitler personally lifted the nationwide curfew so German citizens could enjoy the presumptive victory in the cafés and bars that would carry the broadcast. In the United States, President Franklin Delano Roosevelt invited Louis to the White House—a highly unusual honor for a

Black man at the time—where he gave the boxer encouragement and told him, "Joe, we need muscles like yours to beat Germany."

When the two boxers returned to the ring in sold-out Yankee Stadium, the eyes and especially the ears of the world were on them—it is believed to be the single most listened to radio broadcast in human history, with more than seventy million worldwide tuning in. More than eighty years later, historians still call it the "Fight of the Century," even though it lasted less than one round, with Louis battering Schmeling and knocking him out in just two minutes and four seconds. The American champion would successfully defend his title twenty-five more times in the next eleven years, but it was that 124 seconds that turned Louis into an American icon and hero for the rest of his days. As boxing historian Thomas Hauser wrote in the *Guardian*, it "was the first time that many White Americans openly rooted for a Black man against a White opponent. It was also the first time that many people heard a Black man referred to simply as 'the American.'"

"Louis, who just two years earlier had been viewed by many White Americans as just another Negro fighter, was now embraced by most of the White American public as the appointed defender of their American democracy," wrote William H. Wiggins Jr., professor of folklore and African American studies at Indiana University. "He continued to be accorded respect and admiration by many Americans from all races, creeds, and colors."

During the most active period in the American civil rights movement, the sixties, some other key sports figures impacted spectators, including football's Jim Brown, Olympians John Carlos and Tommie Smith, and of course boxer Muhammad Ali. "The Greatest," Ali was in his heyday equal parts mesmerizing and polarizing, and reviled by many, especially after his conversion to Islam and refusal to fight in the Vietnam War. But he would go on to take his place in history as one of the most beloved American public figures of all time.

★ ★ ★ ★ ★ ★ ★ ★ ★ ★ ★ ★ ★

One of the reasons the civil rights movement went forward was that Black people were able to overcome their fear. And I honestly believe that for many Black Americans, that came from watching Muhammad Ali. He simply refused to be afraid. And being that way, he gave other people courage.

—News anchor Bryant Gumbel in *A People's History of Sports in the United States*

★ ★ ★ ★ ★ ★ ★ ★ ★ ★ ★ ★ ★

In the seventies came Arthur Ashe, who intentionally modeled himself on Robinson to use tennis as a social platform, both here at home and in South Africa, where he was involved early on in the anti–apartheid movement. In a book review of a 2018 biography of the tennis star, the *New York Times* wrote that "[t]ennis was part of a mission to prove Blacks were equal with Whites. To them, mastering tennis and playing it better than most White people would help destroy notions of inherent White superiority ... Ashe belongs on the Mount Rushmore of elite athletes who changed America—put him alongside Muhammad Ali, Jackie Robinson, and Billie Jean King."

In 1984 sports fans were introduced to a new kind of celebrity superstar professional athlete, one whose presence and image and business success transcended all that had come before him, and arguably all who have come since. Michael Jordan changed the way both sports and athletes were marketed, and almost single-handedly elevated the NBA into the much more successful league it is today. He was indispensable in Nike's global success, and as a billionaire who is the all-time highest paid athlete, now co-owns his very own NBA team.

"Think of all the great athletes who came before Michael Jordan," says University of North Carolina professor Matthew Andrews, who specializes in the impact of sports

on American history. "You really had to think about them
in terms of race, whether it was Louis, Owens, Robinson—
that's the burden of the trailblazer, you have to think about
them in terms of race. With Ali in the sixties, everything
is about race. Jordan is this figure who comes along and in
that Gatorade commercial from 1992, who is saying 'I want
to be like Mike.' It's boys and girls, White kids, Brown kids,
Black kids. Jordan is clearly resonating and appealing, in
some ways for the first time in American history, with all
sorts of groups. This has got to have an effect on the way
eighteen years later people were voting for the presidency.
Growing up idolizing a Black athlete, if you're White, has to
have some sort of effect on how you think about politics."

I asked Dr. Kristie to consider a more recent high-profile
athlete, one she had heard of on the news even though she
is still "not a sports fan": 2018 US Women's Open tennis
champion Naomi Osaka, whose mother is Japanese and
father is Afro-Haitian. Japan remains one of the most
racially insular and least diverse developed nations, where
those of mixed ancestry are derisively referred to as *hafu*, a
derogatory bastardization of the English word *half*, meaning "half-breed." As the *Washington Post* reported, "Some
children from mixed race families in Japan often get bul-
lied and demeaned . . . and are chided that they aren't fully
Japanese." Exacerbating this is the fact that linguistic flu-
ency is a culturally integral part of what it means to be

considered "Japanese," and Osaka, whose first language is English and has spent most of her life living and training in the United States, doesn't speak it that well. Yet Japan's sporting pride appears to be a more deeply held conviction than race or language preference, and a country not known for embracing racial diversity quickly claimed her as its own.

"[S]he is being lauded in Japan as the first from the country to win a Grand Slam singles tennis title, which has upstaged most questions about her mixed background," wrote Associated Press reporters Stephen Wade and Mari Yamaguchi. "Japan has embraced the twenty-year-old Osaka . . . But her victory also challenges public attitudes about identity in a homogeneous culture that is being pushed to change." The *New York Times* had a similar perspective in a story titled "In US Open Victory, Naomi Osaka Pushes Japan to Redefine Japanese," writing that "[i]n becoming the first Japanese-born tennis player to win a Grand Slam championship, Ms. Osaka, twenty, is helping to challenge Japan's longstanding sense of racial purity and cultural identity." Megumi Nishikura, co-director of the documentary *Hafu: The Mixed-Race Experience in Japan*, told the *Times*, "Anybody who is able to represent Japan in a public way who is 'hafu' will open Japanese minds and hearts to being more accepting." This is a generalization that could apply equally to pop stars or other celebrities, but one of the most common ways to represent Japan in a public way is by doing it in front of sports fans.

Chicago Cubs star pitcher Yu Darvish was born in Japan to a Japanese mother and Iranian father. Before leaving for the United States, Darvish was considered the best pitcher in Japanese baseball and is wildly beloved in the baseball-crazed nation. Three years before Osaka made tennis history, the *Japan Times* featured Darvish as the most prominent example in an article titled "Biracial athletes making strides in changing Japanese society." The AP reporters noted that "[t]he visibility of mixed-race athletes in Japan is sure to increase as the 2020 Tokyo Olympics approach and the country hunts for competitors in sports where it has little history."

★ ★ ★ ★ ★ ★ ★ ★ ★ ★ ★ ★ ★ ★

We want to live in a world that has a sense of humanity . . . where [we are] judged not by the color of their skin or religious beliefs but by their actions and deeds. Sport might not solve every problem, it's not a panacea, but can sport play that role, can it build a stronger humanity? In my view, unquestionably yes.
—**Sir John Key, former prime minister of New Zealand, speaking in Washington, DC, 2019**

★ ★ ★ ★ ★ ★ ★ ★ ★ ★ ★ ★ ★ ★

Soccer is the most popular sport in the world (cricket is second) and is most widespread geographically in its popularity, played in just about every corner of the globe. For this reason, it is the key game Professor Markovits studies. The University of Michigan academic has examined how sports fandom makes us as more "cosmopolitan," which he defines as having more "respect for strangers and the universal recognition of individuals independent of their cultural or racial background, citizenship, and heritage." He went so far in one study as to make the correlation between the United Kingdom being the first major soccer-loving country to widely embrace the importation of foreign players to its top teams and the fact that today the political representation of ethnic minorities is higher in the British parliament than in the government of any other country in Europe.

"In formerly ethnically homogenous Europe, professional soccer has worked as a unique force for diversity, facilitating the democratic inclusion of immigrants," he writes with his co-author, Professor Lars Rensmann, comparing this directly to Jackie Robinson in America, and finally concluding that ". . . it was American sports that played a vanguard role. . . changes toward more inclusion and diversity in America's sports world regularly preceded and anticipated similarly inclusive changes in other cultural, social, and political spheres . . . the stardom of African

Americans in the sports world, as exemplified by basketball stars like Magic Johnson and Michael Jordan or golf legend Tiger Woods, helped expand the social acceptance of Blacks, and thus constituted the precursors to Colin Powell, Condoleezza Rice, and eventually Barack Obama."

Of course, it would be foolish to actually believe that the "changes toward more inclusion and diversity" have been nearly enough, or that people of color do not continue to suffer excessively in everything from arrest rates to income to opportunities. The tragic choking to death of George Floyd by Minneapolis police was just the latest and highest profile in a long series of continuing reminders that racism and racial injustice are still common in American society. Just two months earlier, Breonna Taylor, a twenty-six-year old Black EMT, was shot eight times and killed by Louisville police in her own apartment. Among many other causes he is involved with, LeBron James spent 2020 waging a high-profile campaign to bring the officers who shot Taylor to justice.

In the wake of Floyd's death, LeBron James partnered with other NBA and WNBA stars to launch More Than a Vote. The non-profit organization aims to leverage social media to inspire Blacks to register and vote, combat voter suppression, and draw attention to any attempts to restrict the franchise of racial minorities. "I'm inspired by the likes of Muhammad Ali, I'm inspired by the Bill Russells and the

Kareem Abdul-Jabbars, the Oscar Robertsons—those guys who stood when the times were even way worse than they are today," James told the *New York Times*, which also noted that the NBA's biggest star, who is immensely popular with fans, has the largest social media following of any American athlete, with over 136 million followers.

The nationwide spring 2020 Black Lives Matter protests sparked by Taylor and Floyd's killings were supported by many prominent athletes across major sports, including James, Michael Jordan, Serena Williams, and reigning Super Bowl champion quarterback Patrick Mahomes. Even major European soccer stars and entire teams demonstrated support for Floyd and the Black Lives Matter movement. In an expansion of national anthem kneeling protests by athletes beyond the NFL and NBA, all players and coaches on both the Yankees and Nationals took a knee before the anthem at the opening game of the 2020 MLB season.

All of this led to some changes within the sports world, though many were long overdue. In one notable better-late-than-never sports example, NASCAR quickly decided to ban the Confederate flag, a highly offensive and racially charged symbol, at its races. NFL Commissioner Roger Goodell issued an apology in which he admitted the league had been wrong in ignoring its players and the Black Lives Matter movement, though many felt he did not go far enough, especially since he left out Colin Kaepernick's name, a

glaring omission. Both the NFL and NBA announced new
league-wide social justice messaging campaigns on playing surfaces and uniforms, including adding "Black Lives
Matter" to all NBA courts and allowing players to wear the
message (among others) instead of their names on jerseys,
something many immediately did as play resumed.

The social justice spotlight shone on the sports world
even helped push decades of efforts by Native American
groups and advocates over the top and got the NFL's
Washington Redskins to finally change their name. Major
college and university sports teams had abandoned ste-
reotyped and racist Native American names and logos
years earlier, but the Redskins had hung on adamantly
and unapologetically, with team owner Daniel Snyder
previously insisting the team would "never" change their
name. While they attempt to rebrand, Snyder's franchise
played the 2020 season using the temporary placeholder
"Washington Football Team."

But in a year that saw major expansions in the use of
spectator sports to address social issues, it was the shooting of Jacob Blake by police in Kenosha, Wisconsin, that
caused an unprecedented response from athletes across
multiple major sports. Blake was shot in the back seven
times while trying to enter his car. Three days later, the
Milwaukee Bucks' players "stunned league officials by organizing Wednesday's boycott, a walkout that had virtually

no precedent in NBA history," according to the *New York Times*. The Bucks refused to take the floor in a post-season playoff game, and their example was quickly followed by the Boston Celtics and Toronto Raptors, leading the league to postpone three playoff games. The boycott movement as a form of high-profile protest cascaded across sports, and three Major League Baseball games and five Major League Soccer games were immediately canceled. In individual sports, tennis phenom Naomi Osaka sat out her semifinal match in a New York tournament. The sentiment spanned many sports and was summed up by LeBron James on Twitter, in all caps: "We demand change. Sick of it."

SPORTS FANS AND WOMEN'S RIGHTS

*T*itle IX is a complex federal civil rights law that prohibits educational institutions receiving federal aid, which includes most institutions of higher education, from excluding participation on the basis of sex. It is not specific to sports but is best known for requiring parity among men's and women's teams at colleges, and as such, providing more opportunities for female students to play competitive sports. Dr. Kristie did not play varsity sports in college, though a decade and half from now, her daughter might. But there's an argument to be made that both Dr. Kristie and her daughter benefit from Title IX because there's an argument to be made that all American women do. The law has resulted in more opportunities for sports fans to see female athletes competing, which in turn, just as with Joe Louis and Jackie Robinson, changes the way fans perceive women.

"Title IX I think is the most important law in our country in the last fifty years," said Christine Brennan at the 2019 Vatican-sponsored "Sport at the Service of Humanity" conference. Brennan, among the nation's most prominent sports journalists, is the recipient of more than a dozen awards, including the inaugural Billie Jean King award in journalism (called "the Billie Award"), and a columnist for *USA Today*, a commentator on ABC News, CNN, *PBS NewsHour*, and NPR, and a bestselling author. "I know there's a lot of competition for that that title, but we are just starting to see the value in terms of leadership for women—congress, senate, women running for president, running our universities, our businesses, our nation. It will change the way this nation is built, run, and led over the next half century. We haven't even begun to see the magnitude of change, it is a tidal wave of Title IX."

★ ★ ★ ★ ★ ★ ★ ★ ★ ★ ★ ★

There's this theory that you can't be what you can't see. Well, when you see an athlete who is a woman of color at the highest level of her game being paid a fair wage, I think that's a role model.
—**Cathy Engelbert, WNBA commissioner, former chair & CEO of Deloitte, speaking at the Vatican's "Sports at the Service of Humanity" conference**

★ ★ ★ ★ ★ ★ ★ ★ ★ ★ ★ ★

Longtime college administrator and former University of Washington president Dr. Mark Emmert agrees, but then again, in his current role as president of the National Collegiate Athletic Association (NCAA), the governing body for high-level collegiate competition, you would expect him to be positive about the social impacts of spectator sports. In this case, I believe he also happens to be right.

While discussing Title IX, Emmert told me, "We are closing in on fifty years, and what I've seen is how people's attitudes toward women's capabilities in society have changed so much just in my lifetime. People today just take it for granted that women are ferocious competitors willing to push themselves as hard physically and mentally as any man. And I think a lot of those perspectives have been shaped and showcased through [watching] sports. Sports led that charge, and as result, no one today thinks that a woman can't be a lawyer or be president. We have women governors all over the country." Emmert is probably a bit overzealous, and while it would be great if he was completely right on this issue, unfortunately, I am sure there are still some people who do not think a woman should be president. But I am also hopeful that there has been real progress, some of it due to sports. At the NCAA, he has promoted the use of higher education to combat sexual assault and violence, focused on LGBTQ+ rights, and pushed for greater diversity among coaches and athletic administrators. Three months after I met with him, the hiring of Callie Brownson as an offensive coach made her the first known full-time female football coach in top-tier Division I. Brownson then quickly moved on to the NFL, first with the Buffalo Bills and currently with the Cleveland Browns, and was the fourth woman on an NFL coaching staff at the end of the 2019-2020 season.

Just one year after Title IX was signed into law, but long before anyone knew how big an impact it would have on sports, a higher profile match in terms of gender was playing out in front of a huge audience. The "Battle of the Sexes" was a historical and unprecedented 1973 sporting event that drew ninety million viewers. It pitted Billie Jean King, the winner of thirty-nine Grand Slam titles and number one ranked women's player in the world, against professional tennis player and outspoken male chauvinist Bobby Riggs. After winning the match, King would become a champion for women's liberation, social equality, and equal pay, and was named *Time* magazine's "Person of the Year," *Sports Illustrated*'s "Sportsman of the Year," and was awarded the Presidential Medal of Freedom, our nation's highest civilian honor. *Sports Illustrated* observed, "She has prominently affected the way 50 percent of society thinks and feels about itself in the vast area of physical exercise," and sportswriter Dave Zirin wrote, "The story of the women's movement is incomplete without mention of Billie Jean King's match against Bobby Riggs."

I have often been asked whether I am a woman or an athlete. The question is absurd. Men are not asked that. I am an athlete. I am a woman.
—**Billie Jean King in her memoir,** *Billie Jean*

Dartmouth College religion professor Randall Balmer, who teaches a class called "Sports, Religion, and Ethics," has investigated the role that sports have historically played as an engine for social change. He told me that, "in all sports there is a moment when the racial barriers are breached. Robinson broke the color barrier, and the next year, Harry Truman desegregated the armed forces. For women, there's Title IX. Another example is Muslims coming into the game, like Kareem Abdul-Jabbar. Muhammad Ali is a great example of that, a very important moment in breaking through barriers of not just racial but religious prejudice."

SPORTS FANS AND RELIGIOUS
AND LGBTQ+ TOLERANCE

ew Alcindor had been a high school and college basketball superstar, leading UCLA to three consecutive
national championships, and remains the only three-time
NCAA finals MVP in history. After turning pro, he led the
Milwaukee Bucks to their first NBA title, after which, like
Muhammad Ali, he very publicly acknowledged his Muslim
faith and became Kareem Abdul–Jabbar. He would win
six championships and set still-standing records for most
points (38,387), most times being named league MVP (six),
and most All-Star team appearances (nineteen). When he
retired he was also the all-time leading rebounder, shot
blocker, and game winner in NBA history.

His popularity never waned, and in addition to having
one of the most impressive sports careers of all time, he
compiled an interesting resumé as an actor, appearing in
multiple television dramas and sitcoms, as well as movies,
where he is remembered best for two extremely different
roles. He was a villainous martial arts opponent against

Bruce Lee in Lee's final film, *Game of Death*, and a co-pilot in the classic absurdist comedy spoof *Airplane!* Meanwhile, he remained vocal and active on issues of both religious and racial intolerance throughout his entire playing and post-playing career and most famously boycotted the 1968 Summer Olympics to protest the treatment of Blacks in America. He later received the nation's highest civilian honor, the Presidential Medal of Freedom—as did Ali and King.

A decade before the color barrier was broken in baseball, Hank Greenberg became the game's first Jewish superstar, drawing plenty of insults and discrimination along with the adoration. Like Robinson, he also had to fight discriminating within baseball, where it is widely believed that teams and owners conspired to keep him from breaking the home run record. He nonetheless became known for his towering home runs and the quiet dignity with which he carried himself and ignored the haters; Greenberg is often credited by historians with improving public perception of Jews. Like Joe Louis, his stardom played out against the ominously growing shadow of Nazi Germany and the prelude to war. In his memoir, he recalled that, "as time went by, I came to feel that if I, as a Jew, hit a home run, I was hitting one against Hitler." When war seemed imminent, he enlisted, and when the Japanese bombed Pearl Harbor, he became the first major leaguer to re-enlist. All told, he lost nearly four full seasons of play but returned to baseball and helped his team win the World Series, eventually securing a place in the Hall of Fame.

The role of sports fandom in increasing religious tolerance in this country is less clear than its impact on the civil rights movement, in part because the same levels of legal segregation did not exist for religious differences and also because there have been far fewer superstar athletes representative of religious minorities here. But studies like those done by Markovits and Rensmann on the general growth of cosmopolitanism among fans include religious tolerance as a positive. In European soccer, where there are far more Muslim players than in the United States, they have observed this more acutely—once, memorably, in Scotland's soccer-obsessed Glasgow, as Markovits and Rensmann wrote: "Nothing illustrates the silent transformation toward a modernized, more inclusive, postreligious and postethnic collective identity more strikingly than this brief conservation between a Glaswegian man and a Muslim immigrant woman: 'What are you?' asks the man, whereupon the woman answers, 'I am Muslim,' to which the man responds, 'I know that you are a Muslim, but are you a Celtic-Muslim or a Rangers-Muslim?'"

While sports and its impact on fans was part of the early progress toward civil rights, women's rights, and arguably religious tolerance, the role of sports in LGBTQ+ rights, while now more positive, was slower. In this instance, society changed first and sports followed belatedly, rather than leading the way. Part of this has been an institutional failure within teams and leagues, but overall the track record is poor, though the evidence suggests that fans may have been willing and ready to accept this diversity before sports was ready to give it to them, given the repeated stories of pleasant surprise athletes have recalled of fan reactions after coming out. The silver lining is that teams, leagues, and spectators are finally catching up to society at large, and sports are now helping to move the needle.

"I don't think I could have come out as a gay athlete thirty years ago and expected to be successful in my sport. My story's indicative of change," Gus Kenworthy told *Time* magazine. Kenworthy is a recently retired professional freeskier who won the silver medal for Team USA at the 2014 Sochi Winter Games. But his sexuality was still a secret in a sport that "oozed machismo," as *Time* put it. Among top skiers, "[h]omophobic taunts were common. *Fag* was a term of ridicule. Bad tricks were dismissed as 'gay.'"

"When you hear language like that getting thrown around, it puts you in a closet even more than you were before," Kenworthy said. So he made a plan, which he later explained to *ESPN the Magazine*: "I didn't want to come out as the silver medalist from Sochi. I wanted to come out as the best freeskier in the world." Fueled by this inspiration he quickly won back-to-back-to-back events in Aspen, Mammoth, and Park City to take the world number-one ranking. True to his plan, he then came out as the first openly gay action-sports champion and high-profile competitor—and proceeded to have the best year of his career, making podium after podium, including two silver medals in the X Games and another at the World Ski Championships.

But his biggest surprise was the public response. Fans expressing support far outweighed those who didn't, and strangers thanked him for his courage and inspiration. An impressed mother named her son Gus after him. Major sponsors backed him, including Procter & Gamble, United Airlines, Visa, and Deloitte. Competitors he had known for years called to apologize for insensitive things they had said in front of him. Now, "[t]hey'll be like 'that's so ga—. . . lame,'" Kenworthy said. "That actually means a lot to me."

He broke his thumb practicing for the 2018 Winter Games in South Korea, but still got satisfaction from all the fan support, telling *People* magazine, "That just makes me feel like I've done something right and it makes me happy that I did it in such a public way. Because in some regards it's your own business, it's not really anybody else's, but I think that the reason that I wanted to do it in a big way

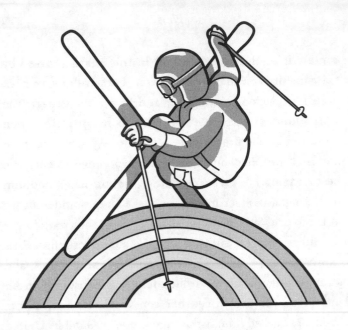

and make a big splash was because it's so unexpected in our sport and in action sports, and I think that the only way to really battle homophobia and battle stereotypes is just by having visibility and being public and open and honest and authentic."

Interestingly, when Kenworthy transitioned to the next phase of his career—acting—and landed a role as Emma Roberts' boyfriend on the single-season-story-arc horror franchise *American Horror Story* for its "1984" season (in 2019), he got pushback from the gay community, as he related in an op-ed for ESPN. "The gay community is the most supportive community in the world and also the quickest to cut you down . . . Some people wanted to know how I was cast as a straight man or if I could play straight. Is that even a question? I spent the first twenty-three years of my life playing a straight man."

Orlando Cruz had a similarly positive experience when he announced to the world that he was gay, the first prominent boxer ever to do so. Cruz, who competed for Puerto Rico as an amateur in the Olympics and then turned pro, amassing twenty-five career wins, was competing at the sport's highest level, a national champion fighting to become world champ. While he publicly stated his goal of becoming the first gay world champion, he lost his title bid for the World Boxing Organization (WBO)'s World Lightweight Championship in the eighth round. According to the *New Yorker*, "When the boxer . . . issued a press release on October 3, 2012, announcing to the world that he is gay, a strange thing happened: nothing. In a sport that still brims with machismo, nobody in Cruz's circle—not his manager, not his trainer, not his sparring partners— treated him any differently, he said recently, over the phone from Florida." In fact, fans began waving rainbow flags and displaying gay pride symbols at his fights.

There have always been high-profile gay players in sports, and some have publicly come out in the past, but in most cases it was after retirement, such as diver Greg

Louganis, a four-time Olympic gold medalist; journeyman baseball player Billy Bean (now MLB's first Ambassador for Inclusion); longtime NBA player John Amaechi; and NFL veterans Kwame Harris and Esera Tuaolo. The notable exceptions were two of the most dominant and success-ful women tennis players of all time, Billie Jean King and Martina Navratilova, who both played after coming out, the latter for twenty-five years through the peak of her career.

"[A] lot of questions they ask about gay athletes, were essentially the same questions they used to ask about us, the Black athletes," said NBA legend Bill Russell, who became the first Black coach in any major US sport with the Boston Celtics in 1966. Russell noted the similarities between sports' impact in the civil rights struggle and prog-ress toward gay rights while speaking at the LBJ Library's Civil Rights Summit in Austin in 2014.

When All-American Michael Sam was selected by the St. Louis Rams out of the University of Missouri in 2014, he became the first openly gay player drafted in NFL his-tory. In four pre-season games, he became the first openly gay player to take the field in an NFL game. He was cut by the Rams at the end of pre-season, briefly signed with the Dallas Cowboys, then moved to the Canadian Football League, where he again made sports history, becoming the first openly gay player to ever play in the CFL. But his career was short-lived—he starred in just one regular season game, missed several others for injury and personal reasons, and abruptly retired. When Jackie Robinson "made the turnstiles click," he disproved concerns about fans finding his race in the game off-putting. Sam never had that opportunity in terms of ticket sales, but supportive fans still voted with their wallets. Interestingly, despite staying in the league only through pre-season, his immediately become the second best-selling rookie jersey in the NFL, and the sixth best overall—an impressive feat when you consider that the NFL has just shy of seventeen hundred players.

In 2013 Boston Celtics center Jason Collins became the first active player in the big four American sports to come out. Major League Soccer (MLS) has had openly gay active players since 2013. More recently, in fall 2018, Tadd Fujikawa—the golfer best known for being, at age fifteen, the youngest player ever to qualify for and play in the US Open, and then as the youngest ever to make the cut in a PGA Tour event—broke new ground once again as the first male pro golfer come out as gay. He did it via his social media account on World Suicide Prevention Day, posting: "Although it's a lot more accepted in our society these days, we still see children, teens, and adults being ridiculed and discriminated against for being the way we are. Some have even taken their lives because of it. As long as those things are still happening, I will continue do my best to bring more awareness of this issue and fight for equality." Afterward, Fujikawa told *Golfweek* reporter Eamon Lynch that he was overwhelmed by the positive response he got from fans and the public.

SPORTS FANS HAVE TO DO BETTER

*D*r. Kristie was genuinely encouraged that fandom had lessened discrimination and increased tolerance, but we both agreed that we were living in the most politically and culturally divisive period either of us could recall in our lives, when hate and White supremacist groups have been on the rise, while former President Donald Trump and other high-level elected officials regularly publicly classified entire nationalities and ethnic groups as criminals. Bullying, exacerbated by social media, remains a major problem. Income inequality, law enforcement inequality, and sentencing inequality have further divided the country.

In a 2019 national telephone survey, author and professor Michael Serazio and his colleagues found that half the population felt strongly that politics and sports should not mix, while only 20 percent thought they should. According to Serazio, more Americans believe that God has an active role in determining who wins a game than the idea that sports and politics should intertwine.

Yet they are intertwined. There is a long tradition of winning teams of all sorts receiving White House invites, and this is always political, but under the Trump administration it became contentious, and several athletes refused to accept. Around the world, politicians are expected and in some cases required to attend major sporting events or risk drawing negative media attention by their absence, especially in soccer's World Cup. More than ever, in today's digital information age, sports and politics are inseparable. The results can be good, bad, or simply informative.

When Trump used his office to take to Twitter to condemn and insult professional athletes—in Trump's case almost exclusively Black professional athletes—it showed a very large swath of the public a side of him they might not otherwise have seen. When the same president attended a World Series game in October 2019 and was roundly booed by the sold-out crowd in the nation's capital—booed lengthily along with chants of "lock him up"—it showed a reaction to Trump that many might not have otherwise seen. When high profile athletes in the NBA, NFL, and other leagues demonstrate their support for causes like #BlackLivesMatter, it brings a new level of media and audience attention to those very real issues.

"There was a day when we saw sports as an escape. The sports section would take you someplace that the A section of the newspaper did not," said *USA Today* columnist

Christine Brennan. "Of course, what has happened now, and I think it's a good thing, is that the sports section is no longer an escape, it is a mirror of our society. When you grab that sports section, so many of those pages and stories and headlines you read, whether it's in print or online, those stories are about so much more than sports." Given that for many viewers, sports news on TV is news on TV, period, Brennan's point is relevant, and she feels strongly about it. I agree with her. "Knowledge is power. Sports takes us to national conversations, and frankly I think it helps us with those conversations. The Larry Nassar USA Gymnastics horrors, well a whole different audience was exposed to that because it was about sports, and of course, about so much more than sports. But those reading it might never have read about those issues in another forum."

Kareem Abdul-Jabbar has remained a prominent figure in conversations about race and religion since his earliest playing days, and in 2018 he wrote an opinion column for London's the *Guardian* noting the real importance of all his many records: "The even greater significance those records had to me then, and has to me even more now, is in providing a platform to keep the discussion of social inequalities—whether racial, gender-related, or economic—alive and vibrant so that we may come together as a nation and fix them . . . whatever happens in sports regarding race, plays out on the national stage. Right now, sports may be the best hope for change regarding racial disparity because it has the best chance of informing White Americans of that disparity and motivating them to act."

University of North Carolina history professor Matthew Andrews teaches classes such as "Sport and American History," "Baseball and American History," and a sports and civil rights research seminar. I got him on the phone and asked him his views on the impact of sports on fans. "You're asking the exact types of questions I try to figure out in my sports history class: to what extent do these athletes like Jackie Robinson, Joe Louis, Muhammed Ali, Colin Kaepernick have an effect on larger society?" He uses Ali's famous protest of the war in Vietnam as an example of how difficult it is to isolate or prove causal factors when it comes to history, acknowledging that Ali brought much attention to the issue, but that attention is not the same as resolution: "Yes, education and illuminating issues and problems is part of the process of change. But what changes more minds about Vietnam: Ali's refusal to be inducted or America seeing the Tet Offensive on television?" In this case, it took a change of public opinion about the justness of the conflict—and many years to pass—before acceptance of the boxer's political stance, which originally was widely rejected.

Andrews told me, "When Ali died, the tributes to him were almost unanimously popular; he was talked about as a man of principle, and basically the general argument was that Ali was right and the people who opposed him were wrong. I absolutely see that as evidence of positive change in this country, that we're willing to praise someone who questioned American foreign policy in a way that we weren't as a nation in the sixties. So, I would certainly answer yes, that the way we celebrate these athletes now is indicative of some sort of positive change."

Today's athletes continue to try and change hearts and minds, starting with their fans, and thanks to the digital age, athletes are able to speak to audiences directly and faster. Attorney and former NFL commissioner Paul Tagliabue is now chairman of the Ross Initiative in Sports for Equality (RISE), a national nonprofit that educates and empowers the sports community to eliminate racial discrimination, champion social justice, and improve race relations. Many of their initiatives are focused on the hot-button issues of policing in low-income neighborhoods. Tagliabue spoke about this at the Sports at the Service of Humanity Conference:

> Sports leagues are in the process of reinventing themselves. They are moving into spaces that have to do with major issues in society. The athletes in particular are moving beyond being athletes and becoming educators, leaders, facilitators on societal

issues. I think the transformation is just beginning, and if you look at it there are three reasons: The athletes themselves have grown in up in segments of society which are suffering, and it gets into issues of income inequality, law enforcement profiling, a lot of issues the athletes know about because they grew up in those communities and they want to have voice to rectify those injustices. Secondly, it's resources. When I started working on the NFL staff in 1969, the typical player might be making $35,000. Today it might be $3.5 million and lots of them are making ten million or more. The athletes have resources, they can have staff, they can have outlets, they can partner with other programs and bring resources to the table. The third thing is the platforms that are available. When I left as commissioner there were no smartphones. There was no Facebook. We were dealing with traditional media, not what's out there creating this interconnected society. When you put those three things together, there is tremendous potential for professional athletes, coaches, and other leaders in professional sports to have impact on societal issues that did not exist earlier.

Take the case of George Zimmerman, found not guilty in the 2012 killing of unarmed Black teen Trayvon Martin, a high school student shot on the street while visiting his father in Sanford, Florida, causing large public rallies in multiple cities. Members of the closest NBA team, the Miami Heat, joined the discussion on social media. Superstars LeBron James, Chris Bosh, and Dwyane Wade also showed up on the court wearing hoodies, the garment that apparently had made the Florida teen "suspicious" to Zimmerman.

Ever since, a wave of athletes have been involved in the #BlackLivesMatter movement and other protests against the mistreatment of Black and Latino citizens by law enforcement in this country. Another widely covered incident occurred when New York City police officers used a chokehold on Eric Garner, who died an hour later. In the video of the arrest, which went viral, Garner calls out "I can't breathe" eleven times, and this became a catch phrase for protesters—including the biggest NBA star, LeBron James, who wore a T-shirt emblazoned with the words as a visual protest. He was joined by several other players, including Derrick Rose and Kyrie Irving. WNBA players staged similar on-court protests following two other police killings in 2016, Alton Sterling in Baton Rouge, Louisiana, and Philando Castile in Minnesota.

Four years later, another killing of a Black man by police in Minnesota, George Floyd, would result in an even bigger wave of national protests. This time teams and leagues,

here and abroad, would join the voices of individual athletes. "Amid recent protests over the police killing of George
Floyd and racism reckoning, sports leagues, athletes, and
brands—inclined to project an apolitical image—are coming out in an unprecedented, full-throated defense of protests against racism and injustice," wrote Insider.com's
Ellen Cranley (previously *Business Insider*). "The protests
have opened the floodgates of athletes, leagues, and brands
to speak out after years of resistance and hesitation, paint-
ing a potential future for athletes as activists."

That has certainly been the case for the NBA's biggest
star, LeBron James. When conservative Fox News host
Laura Ingraham suggested in February 2018 that instead
of publicly discussing his political opinions, which is one
America's most sacred rights, he should "shut up and
dribble," the remark took on a life of its own. Not long
after, the Showtime network partnered with James, as
executive producer, to produce a three-part documentary series about the changing role of athletes in today's
political environment—not coincidentally titled *Shut Up
and Dribble*. The series received an Emmy nomination and
examined the changing role of Black athletes in today's cultural and political environments. One installment focused
on early basketball standouts who impacted the world off
the court. These included longtime author, writer, activist,

and multiple NBA record-setter Kareem Abdul-Jabbar and Bill Russell, an NBA superstar, the first Black head coach in any North American professional sport, and a Civil Rights activist who was awarded the Presidential Medal of Freedom.

★ ★ ★ ★ ★ ★ ★ ★ ★ ★ ★ ★ ★

I am deeply disappointed by the tone of the comments made by the President on Friday. I am proud to be associated with so many players who make such tremendous contributions in positively impacting our communities. Their efforts, both on and off the field, help bring people together and make our community stronger. There is no greater unifier in this country than sports, and unfortunately, nothing more divisive than politics.
—New England Patriots owner Robert Kraft
in the *New York Times*

★ ★ ★ ★ ★ ★ ★ ★ ★ ★ ★ ★ ★

The highest profile protest was NFL quarterback Colin Kaepernick's refusal to stand for the national anthem in response to the treatment of American Blacks by police. It is believed by many to have cost him his playing career, and drew the direct personal anger of then-President Trump in

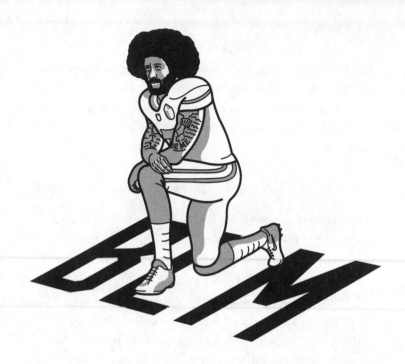

a series of tweets, some of which urged teams to fire protesters. This was part of the president's larger wave of angry
tweets aimed at predominantly Black athletes, including
NBA star Steph Curry, after he became the first of many
spotlight athletes to publicly refuse an invitation to the
White House in protest.

A sizable number of fans are still deeply angered by the
national anthem protests, but far less than when he began.
In September 2016, two weeks after the first pre-season

protest, a whopping 72 percent of the American public—nearly three-quarters—thought the quarterback's actions were unpatriotic. Less than two years later, the tables had turned. A major national Quinnipiac University poll showed that by mid-2018, a majority of Americans now believed the protests were not unpatriotic. That is a landslide shift, and while a few other national polls in 2018 had conflicting split results, all the numbers had substantially changed in favor of the protestors. Then–Miami Dolphins star receiver Kenny Stills continued one of the longest kneeling protest streaks in the league into the 2018 season, and he told reporters after opening day how much had changed in just two years: "There's been a huge difference between when we first started protesting and now, a lot of people reaching out and supporting us."

We will not stand for the injustice that has plagued people of color in this country. Out of love for our country and in honor of the sacrifices made on our behalf, we unite to oppose those that would deny our most basic freedoms.
—Prepared statement issued by
the NFL's Seattle Seahawks

Likewise, NFL ratings, which had been in decline, especially right after the protests began—also likely related to the league's concussion problems—sharply rebounded for the 2018 season. On opening weekend, with the protests still ongoing, CBS had its most-watched debut game in twenty years, with a stunning 29 percent increase over the previous season, while both the games that Fox broadcast had notable annual increases, reversing the downward trend. *USA Today* pointed out that virtually all scheduled television is in decline due to the rise of streaming services (Hulu, Netflix, Amazon Prime Video, etc.) and alternate programming, so even just holding steady is considered a success. The NFL actually gained followers.

This trend continued into 2019, when ratings returned to their 2016 high, gaining 3 percent over the previous year through the first six weeks of the season, and 9 percent overall since the 2017 low, prompting the *Hollywood Reporter* to write, "Like a quarterback shrugging off a sack, the NFL is brushing off doubts about its ratings supremacy among US TV viewers . . . now, as ratings for other programming keep declining, the audience for the NFL is rising."

In the fall of 2018, when Nike made the surprise announcement that they had not only chosen to extend Kaepernick's endorsement contract, but would use the

quarterback—who had not played a down in two years—
as a face of the thirtieth anniversary of the brand's world
famous "Just Do It" marketing campaign (along with
LeBron James and Serena Williams), passions were reig-
nited. Anti-protest protesters burned Nike gear, displaying
the videos on social media, and threatened boycotts, while
supporters rushed to buy more Swooshes. Trump again
took to Twitter, this time to ask "What was Nike thinking?"
but within forty-eight hours after the ad debuted, online
sales skyrocketed and were up 31 percent over the same
period the year before.

If voting with their wallets showed fans were in support
of the protests, their message was loud and clear: during the
next two weeks, the women's model of the Kaepernick jersey
sold out completely and overall Nike sales climbed 61 percent. Trump tweeted again, this time falsely claiming that
"Nike is getting absolutely killed with anger and boycotts,"
even as its stock price surged 7 percent to an all-time high.
CNBC reported that the campaign had drawn a record number of likes to Nike's social media platforms, while analysts
at financial services firm Canaccord Genuity surveyed the
public on the ad campaign and concluded that despite pushback from vocal anti-protest consumers, most "overwhelmingly" supported it, and more than twice as many said they
would "absolutely buy more Nike" after seeing the ad.

★ ★ ★ ★ ★ ★ ★ ★ ★ ★ ★ ★

**Kaepernick's return could be a ratings bonanza.
Interest in, and support for, Kaepernick remains
so strong that his Nike ads are credited with
boosting the company's stock price.
—*Washington Post* opinion columnist Max Boot**

★ ★ ★ ★ ★ ★ ★ ★ ★ ★ ★ ★

New Yorker staff writer Jelani Cobb observed that, "Improbably, Colin Kaepernick's social stature has only grown since his departure from the NFL. In 2017, he was named *GQ*'s Citizen of the Year, and, in 2018 won Amnesty International's Ambassador of Conscience Award. During a time in which he never set foot on the field, his No. 7 jersey outsold those of most active players." Shortly after the 2018 NFL season began, Harvard University announced that it would bestow the W.E.B. Du Bois Medal on Kaepernick. The medal honors recipients "in recognition of their contributions to African and African American culture and the life of the mind."

SPORTS FANS AND WORLD PEACE

r. Kristie and I took a late lunch break, avoiding the peak twelve-to-one window in which on-mountain restaurants at ski resorts are typically jammed. Hungry and a bit weary, we removed our jackets and sat down, settling in for a prolonged break. Having bummed out Dr. Kristie with some of the unpleasant realities of inequality and injustice in our nation, I thought she deserved some more pleasant lunch conversation: world peace. Of course, like just about every social issue that intersects with sports fandom, the end game remains unattained, but in this case, there are some really concrete advances and improvements that I find very inspirational.

"Have you ever seen the movie *Invictus* with Matt Damon and Morgan Freeman? It's about rugby."

Dr. Kristie hadn't seen it, but I just had. "It's a true story about sports and much more," I said.

To fully appreciate the role of sports fandom in the march toward world peace one must consider post-apartheid

South Africa, known as "the South African Miracle." British journalist John Carlin, who lived in and covered South Africa for years, wrote, "No country has ever shepherded itself from tyranny to democracy more ably, and humanely."

★ ★ ★ ★ ★ ★ ★ ★ ★ ★ ★ ★ ★

It has the power to inspire. It has the power to unite people in a way that little else does . . . Sport can create hope where once there was only despair. It is more powerful than government in breaking down racial barriers. It laughs in the face of all types of discrimination.
—South African president and Nobel Peace Prize recipient Nelson Mandela

★ ★ ★ ★ ★ ★ ★ ★ ★ ★ ★ ★ ★

Political commentator and author Justice Malala wrote in the *Guardian*, "If there is one thing South Africans agree on, it is that our country is a far better place than the monstrosity it was before 1994. The fruits of freedom are numerous and real for many of us: a country where we walk proudly, without fear; a full citizenship of the world; a democratic dispensation and constitution to be proud of."

Many historians maintain that the largely peaceful change in regime and racial relations in South Africa was the fastest and most dramatic in human history. When apartheid ended, only half the population had electricity—now it's more than 85 percent. The murder rate, once among the highest anywhere in the world, has dropped by well over half, and millions more citizens live in modern houses. Black South Africans account for more than three-quarters of new business startups, and the percentage of Blacks graduating from college has more than doubled.

It is a truly remarkable story, one for which Mandela is rightfully given much of the credit, but one that likely could not have transpired as it did without White South Africa's obsession with rugby—by far their favorite sport. Immediately after Mandela's election, the hotly divided nation teetered on the brink of violent civil war and at one point a military coup seemed likely, but these worries were erased—with the help of sports.

The story of how Mandela used rugby, on par with religion amongst a group for whom religion was serious business, to unify the nation is best told in John Carlin's excellent book *Playing the Enemy: Nelson Mandela and the Game that Made a Nation*, the basis for *Invictus*. Years before his election, while still in prison, Mandela laid out his detailed plan to use rugby fandom as a bridge to bring Blacks and Whites together, a plan that succeeded beyond expectations, and is the starkest example of sports fandom as a tool for peace, a friend of tolerance, and an enemy of racism.

Here is the short version of South Africa's real-life rugby fairy tale: The Springboks, named for a type of African antelope, were the nation's national team and once considered a rugby powerhouse, but because of international boycotts against apartheid, for years they had not been allowed to travel abroad to play, even for the once-every-four-years World Cup, and no one would come to South Africa for matches. Mandela and his political party, the African National Congress (ANC), had successfully used their voice throughout the world to encourage boycotts and international protests in order to bring pressure on the government, and that included rugby. When the potential for free elections finally appeared on the horizon, Mandela, who was negotiating toward a change of power with then-President F.W. de Klerk, offered to give rugby back and bring the 1995 World Cup to South Africa if the elections could go on. This was a powerful bargaining chip, and it worked, but that is only half the story.

The other half is that the Black majority of South Africans loathed rugby, saw it as what it was, a White man's game, and furthermore, detested the Springboks, which they considered a symbol of apartheid, on equal footing with the racist national anthem. Once elected, Mandela's second imposing challenge was getting Blacks to switch gears and support the team as a way to unify the country. He pleaded, cajoled, and gave endless speeches, but it remained a tough sell. Yet eventually, he was convincing. Still, Mandela was under heavy pressure from his own supporters to change the name of the team and the symbol, which he refused to do, and to replace the national anthem with a new one. Instead a second anthem was written, and they were both performed. (Interestingly, in South Africa, the president is the only spectator allowed to place his hand over his heart during the performance of the anthem.) As Desmond Tutu explained, Mandela embraced his enemies and gave them back their humanity precisely by not taking away their passions as punishment. The team kept its name but got a catchy new slogan that was widely displayed: "One Team, One Country."

The effort was helped tremendously by the Springboks themselves, who were underdogs to several teams, yet miraculously made it to the final game against the number-one squad, heavily favored New Zealand. When Mandela, whom many Whites had considered a criminal and a threat not just to their way of life but to their very lives, walked out onto the field in his own Springboks hat and jersey—sporting the number of team captain Francois Pienaar—the crowd went wild. White South Africans did not merely accept him; they erupted into foot-stomping chants of "Nelson! Nelson!" that rocked the stadium and shocked outside observers. Until joining them as a fan of rugby, Mandela and most of the crowd had been mortal enemies, and that seemed to change before the first whistle blew. When the Springboks won in Cinderella-story fashion, there were massive celebrations nationwide by fans of all colors, and Carlin cites numerous news reports from affluent enclaves in different cities where "White matrons were shedding generations of prejudice and restraint and hugging their Black housekeepers, dancing with them on the leafy streets of prim neighborhoods."

I've been to every major sporting event in the world, and it's hard to explain just how intense this was. When he came out on the field, the chanting of "Nelson! Nelson!" just went on and on. I didn't know exactly what it was at the time, but it was immediately clear that something fundamental in that country had changed completely in that instant.

—Former sportscaster Chad Clark, as told to the author

Archbishop Tutu, a Nobel Peace Prize winner like Mandela, summed it up best: "If you had predicted just a year—just months—earlier that people would be dancing in the streets of Soweto to celebrate a Springbok victory, most people would have said, 'You've been sitting in the South African sun too long, and it's affected your brain.' That match did for us what speeches of politicians or archbishops could not do. It galvanized us, it made us realize that it was actually possible for us to be on the same side. It said it is actually possible for us to become one nation."

In *Playing the Enemy*, Carlin goes to great length to document how the Springbok players themselves began mostly as apolitical middle- and working-class Whites who were cut off from much international opinion about their country and never fully realized that the political system they lived under was detested elsewhere. Pienaar, the hero Springbok captain played by Matt Damon in the film version, quickly became a highly visible face of the young Whites in a new South Africa. When he told his personal story to the *Guardian,* the paper began its profile this way: "Among certain White communities in apartheid South Africa, it was taken for granted that Nelson Mandela was a terrorist who must remain behind bars. That was drummed into the young Francois Pienaar, who would one day welcome Mandela to his wedding and name him as godfather to his two sons." It was a sea change.

Even Mandela, one of the greatest statesmen in history, underestimated the power of fandom. He had been a boxer,

and like most South African Blacks of his era, his spectator
sport was soccer. He hated rugby, and before his election, he
did not understand the game. He chose it merely as a tool, a
means to an end. One of the reasons his strategy worked so
well, though, speaks to the particular power of sports: once
exposed, many Blacks, including Mandela himself, fell for
rugby and against all expectations became avid fans.

After I finished my story, Dr. Kristie told me she was
going to watch the movie. "Wow. That's pretty amazing,"
she said.

"I've got another one for you. Have you ever seen *Rocky
IV*? I love the Rocky movies but it's probably the worst
one. Well, second worst. They hit rock bottom with *Rocky
V*. Then it got better again. But anyway there is something
worth remembering about *Rocky IV*."

In *Rocky IV*, fiction's most famous pugilist travels to the
USSR at the height of the Cold War (1985) to battle Drago, a
half-human, half–lab experiment who combines our worst
fears of the era's Russians with the darkest side of "sports
medicine." Drago is a huge, cold, unbeatable man-robot
who has just killed Rocky's close friend, trainer, and con-
fidant—and a longtime heavyweight world champion—
Apollo Creed. Rocky goes to Russia for revenge, but instead
finds himself an unlikely "diplomat," handling himself so
impressively in the ring that he wins over the entirely par-
tisan crowd, which, despite the imminent threat of their

KGB watch dogs, erupts into cheers of "USA! USA!" much to the chagrin of their Communist overlords. The notion of our fierce enemies suddenly tossing aside years of deeply held beliefs over a spectator sports exhibition and cheering for America seems implausible to the point of ridiculousness, and of course, it's all made up. But it actually happened in 2002 when Iranian soccer fans chanted, "we love America" and "long live freedom" from the stands during their national team's World Cup campaign. That was no screenwriter's fantasy and it boggles the mind. Think about it: Iranian fans cheering "we love America."

* * * * * * * * * * * *

**When I watch a match on the TV for our national team, I do not ask if this player or that is a Sunni or a Shiite—I only care about the results.
—Eighteen-year-old soccer fan Mahmood Abed, who sells sunglasses on the street in Baghdad, as told to *NBC News***

* * * * * * * * * * * *

Inspired by Iran's national team and its march to qualify for the World Cup, this eight-year precursor to the Arab Spring—that unfortunately short-lived series of progressive revolutions and regime change across the Middle

East—has become known as the "football revolution." In his bestselling 2004 globalization treatise *How Soccer Explains the World*, Franklin Foer predicted, "When future historians write about the transformation of the Middle East, they will likely wax lyrical about this moment . . . Like the Boston Tea Party, it will likely go down as the moment when the people first realized that they could challenge their tyrannical rulers. For the Iranians, the event has served as the model uprising, so much so that every subsequent high stakes World Cup qualifying match has led Iranians into the streets."

Foer traces this thread of soccer-inspired political change at least back to Spain under the oppressive rule of military dictator General Francisco Franco, who took power after leading his party to victory in the Spanish Civil War. Franco's opposition came from the Barcelona-centered Catalan resistance movement, and the city's storied soccer team, nicknamed Barca, beloved not just in Spain, but one of the most admired in the entire world, became a hotbed of openly anti-Franco sentiment in the otherwise totalitarian regime. "Its fans like to brag that their stadium gave them a space to vent their outrage against the regime," writes Foer. "Emboldened by a hundred thousand people chanting in unison, safety in numbers, fans seized the opportunity to scream things that could never be said, even furtively, on the street or in the café" due to the ubiquitous secret police.

"This is a common enough phenomenon," Foer adds. "There's a long history of resistance movements igniting in the soccer stadium." He calls this simmering fuse within the stadium, the "sportive ground zero," and cites numerous other examples of sports fan–supported revolts against dictatorships, including Milošević's Serbia, Ceaușescu's Romania, and Stroessner's Paraguay.

The "football revolution" resulted in a more liberal, modern, and, frankly, Westernized Iranian fan, and is also viewed by historians as a landmark advance for women's rights in the region. The team's Brazilian coach—the first foreigner to ever lead the national team—helped set the tone, not only as a beloved outsider, but as one patrolling the sideline in jacket and tie—"European" garb long rejected by the conservative religious leaders. After each victory, celebrants took to the streets of Tehran without regard for traditional restrictions, publicly dancing, drinking alcohol, and listening to Western popular music. Unusually, both sexes mingled together at the festivities, but even more shocking were the many women who took off their hijabs and partied with their heads heretically exposed.

The biggest moment came three days after the final qualifying win overseas against Australia, the game that gave Iran its first trip to the World Cup since the revolution against the Shah over three decades earlier. When the team came home, the government threw them an official

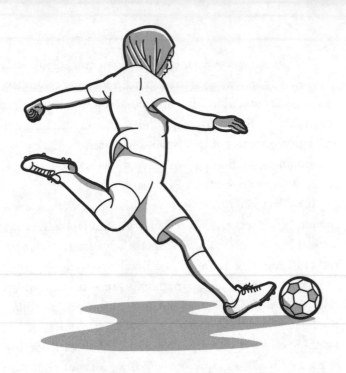

celebration in the city's soccer stadium—some things are the same in sports everywhere—but as was Iranian tradition, the event was for men only. This time, however, the women fans didn't take the discrimination sitting down. Instead, thousands marched on the stadium shouting, "Aren't we part of this nation, too? We want to celebrate. We aren't ants." Some were let through, but not enough, so they stormed the gates, forced their way past police, and joined the celebration.

By Iran's next go at the World Cup, the newfound freedoms that fans expressed grew beyond dancing and drinking and into a more anti-government sentiment. Noting the growing impact of soccer fandom on the entire region, the *New York Times* concluded that, "The game probably matters even more in Iran, a state gripped in recent years by what has been called 'a soccer revolution.' . . . Thousands of women broke into the stadium to join the celebrations, some removed their veils, and at street parties across the country, men and women danced and kissed, defying government warnings and clerical taboos."

In 2007 neighboring Iraq stunned soccer pundits by winning the Asian Cup, the continent's most prestigious tournament. CNN called it "the biggest prize in the country's sporting history." The victory was the climax of a longer road, with unprecedented community **bonding** and national solidarity en route to the final. As CNN reported, "In a country that was fracturing along religious and ethnic lines, its soccer stars had begun to offer an example of how Iraqis could work together. A team of Sunnis, Shiites, and Kurds could easily have been divided, just like their countrymen. But the players agreed to leave religion at the door. They found a way to unite. Not only that, they inspired. 'People's support for us started increasing. We started seeing that we are unifying the people,' Sadir [a player] said." To cement the team's public example of cooperative diversity, the coach halted the tradition of players praying together in their respective groups before the game or at halftime, something Middle Eastern teams regularly did.

After the upset win, Iraqis took to the streets in celebration, a scene CNN Senior International Correspondent Arwa Damon would later call one of her best moments in reporting: "I'm still smiling now as I remember it. It was just such a rare and unique moment for that country that has been through so much."

In 2017 international soccer federation officials deemed it safe to allow the Iraqi national team to play its first international match in years on home soil, against Jordan, in the city of Basra. The religiously diverse team had not forgotten the positive impact they had in 2007 and continued its mission to promote togetherness. As NBC News proclaimed, "Iraq's national soccer team aims to prove to ISIS that 'Nothing Can Divide Us,'" adding "For many Iraqis, the ethnically and religiously mixed team is living, breathing proof that ISIS' philosophy has no place in the country." A Baghdad barber told CBS, "The Iraqi team represents all Iraqis. It doesn't represent Sunnis or Shiites, neither Arabs, Kurds, Muslims, nor Christians."

In 2016 James M. Dorsey released his book, *The Turbulent World of Middle Eastern Soccer,* and spoke about the Arab Spring at the Washington Institute for Near East Policy, echoing Foer's prediction a decade earlier. "The soccer pitch can also be a barometer of future events. In Jordan, statements openly critical of the royal family's corruption first gained notoriety on the soccer field. And at Saudi soccer matches, many princes are booed, pelted with various objects, and sometimes forced off the pitch entirely. Last year's removal of the head of the Saudi Arabian Football Federation was perhaps the first time a royal family member was forced to resign from a post due to public pressure." But more concretely, he concluded that, "Over the past several years, soccer fields across the Middle East and North Africa have become battlegrounds for political, gender, and labor rights, as well as issues of national, ideological, and ethnic identity."

Dorsey is hardly alone in this belief. In an academic article titled "From football riot to revolution. The political role of football in the Arab world," University of Oslo social anthropologist Dag Tuastad finds that, "In the Arab world, ideological resistance of supporters during football matches have coalesced with another rebellion, of youth breaking the chains of patriarchal power. The political implication of this social process is tremendous . . . As football is a primary medium through which youth autonomy could be experienced, football has a seismic political potential . . . The supporters have initiated struggles crucially affecting political developments in their countries."

English journalist and author James Montague argues that soccer fans are as passionate in the Middle East as in better-known hotbeds of the game's obsession such as South America, and noted that "... every Friday, from Aden to Aleppo, millions of fans leave the mosque and head straight for their local football club. In the absence of true democracy and a genuine public space, the terraces [stands in a soccer stadium] provide a forum for dissent." In the introduction to his book *When Friday Comes: Football, War, and Revolution in the Middle East,* Montague asserts that "In the Middle East there was the mosque and the terrace and little in between." He pointedly notes that while an enormous amount of study has gone into how religion affects the region, virtually no attention has been given to sport, attributing this to "a misguided idea that sport and politics are separate entities. Football is politics the same way music is politics, or art, or film. It is an expression of the soul with a tribal beat. But yet football played its role—in some countries a vital role—in the greatest political upheaval to affect the region since the end of colonial rule."

Egypt was the most visible tip of the spear in the Arab Spring, overthrowing longtime dictator Hosni Mubarak, who had "enjoyed near absolute power for three decades," according to the *Telegraph.* During his thirty-year rule, he had survived ten attempts on his life, but in 2011 the Egyptian people had had enough and, led by the most ardent soccer fans—the "ultras,' or die-hard fan clubs— they rebelled.

"[I]n Egypt people fought back. Not on the streets, but first in the stadiums. Then outside the stadiums. And then on the streets. For three years the ultra groups of Egypt's biggest clubs grew more anti-regime with every beating and arrest. Yet they couldn't be controlled. When the dam burst on 25 January 2011, the ultras were on the front line," writes Montague, who concludes that, "Football didn't cause the Arab Spring. The neglect, humiliation and abuse of the poor and the young did. But in the game many found a voice that would not be heard by any other means . . ." Sports fans are a voice that have been heard, loud and clear, all over the world.

SPORTS, FANS, AND DIPLOMACY

*A*s our day on the slopes progressed, Dr. Kristie and I got to talking about the Winter Olympics. She likes the skiing events in particular. So do I.

"Have you ever read the Olympic Charter?" I asked her.

"No, I have not!"

"There is surprisingly little about sports in there. It's mostly about what the authors think sports embodies, values and ideals. Have you ever read the United Nations Charter?"

"No, again!"

"Same thing. Very little about politics or nations, more about ideals. In fact the language is very similar. Maybe that's why the two organizations have an ongoing partnership. May I tell you a story?" Dr. Kristie had been listening to me all day, but I worried I was pushing my luck, so before she could stop me, I started right in.

The West African nation of Côte d'Ivoire (Ivory Coast) has long been an unstable and divided country. In less than twenty years, it had endured a military coup and two different civil wars. UN peacekeepers, looking for a way to bridge that divide at the local level, came upon the idea of organizing a soccer game, with each team comprised of a mix of players from opposing factions. It was a twist on neuropsychologist Jay Van Bavel's minimal group theory experiments, but with real teams playing an actual sport. It was novel, generated a lot of local interest, and was heavily attended by curious onlookers from both groups.

The story I was relaying to Dr. Kristie was one told to me by Andrea Talentino, who taught political science at Nazareth College and specializes in military intervention and civil conflict. She chaired an interdisciplinary academic conference on sports that I attended and described what happened in the Ivory Coast when the rest of the citizenry—the fans—saw those groups "wearing the same jerseys and cooperating. They were amazed." As a result, the games continued, the program ran for five more years, and Talentino described it as one of the most sustained, comprehensive, and successful such efforts by the UN to leverage sports. "Sport is universal. Whether it's sub–Saharan Africa or the West, it's everybody. Sports are a meeting place where ignorance and intolerance can be overcome. That's where the value lies."

★ ★ ★ ★ ★ ★ ★ ★ ★ ★ ★ ★

We believe that:
Sport has the power to celebrate our common humanity,
regardless of faith, race, culture, beliefs,
gender, and ability.
Sport can bring us together—to meet one another across
borders and boundaries, to learn to compete as friends, to
respect and trust one another even in opposition.
**—From the Preamble to the Declaration of Principles
for the Sport at the Service of Humanity initiative**

★ ★ ★ ★ ★ ★ ★ ★ ★ ★ ★ ★

The United Nations has identified sports "as a tool for development and peace" and created an entire department devoted to it. The United Nations has noted that the positive attributes of sports could help in accomplishing its mission in no fewer than a dozen areas: sustainable human development, economic development, peace, health, education, the environment, volunteerism, communication, social mobilization, partnerships, HIV/AIDS, and human rights.

Similar logic was at work in October 2016 when Pope Francis launched the Sport at the Service of Humanity (SSH) initiative. The Vatican describes this as the "only global sport and multi-faith movement." Pope Francis, from Argentina, is known to be a serious soccer fan, supporting both his home club of San Lorenzo and the Argentinean national team.

Diplomacy and sports have been linked for a long time. Diplomacy has always used sports.
—**Former US Ambassador and current Cubs fan Peter DeShazo, as told to the author**

The 2018 Summit meeting in Singapore between the leaders of United States and North Korea, may not amount to much—if anything-—in the long run. But just the fact that there were talks at all was progress, progress directly related to spectator sports. Prior to the 2018 Winter Olympic Games, no US president had ever set foot on North Korean soil or met with the nation's leader, and prior to that, conversations between the two countries consisted mainly of threats—often on Twitter—of annihilation or conquest of one another by the bombastic and unpredictable leaders of the time. The Olympics opened the door to diplomacy and were the catalyst for the talks.

"Many considered it an impossible dream to have an Olympics of peace, in which North Korea would participate and the two Koreas would form a joint team," said South Korea's President Moon Jae-in, who saw the games as a key tool to engage reclusive North Korea and bring them back to the negotiating table regarding its nuclear and ballistic missile program. The mood of the 2018 Winter Olympic Games, held in South Korea, were set right at the outset, with North Korea and South Korea marching under one flag in the opening ceremonies, and in some cases fielding unified teams—a far cry from the 1988 Sydney Games in which North Korea stayed home after being found culpable in the terrorist bombing of a South Korean passenger jet that killed all 115 passengers and crew on board.

As the *New York Times* reported, "Whereas recent Olympic Games have sought to set politics aside, the strategic subtext of the event in Pyeongchang has been unavoidable. Kim Yo-jong, the younger sister of Kim Jong-un, North Korea's leader, was sitting at the opening ceremony closely behind Vice President Mike Pence, who led the American delegation." Neither leader attended, but it was these right-hand men and women who started the ball rolling, a process that would culminate in the historic meeting in Singapore.

"What you're seeing in Korea can be traced all the way back to the ancient Greeks," Carlos Tigreros told me.

When I spoke with him, Tigreros was beginning a second career in the State Department's Foreign Service after five years serving in the navy as a nuclear engineer, mostly in the South China Sea, followed by a masters in globalization studies. He seemed genuinely surprised that I even raised the question of the importance of sports fandom in world affairs, as if the connection were obvious. He even argued that it was Jong-un's famous love of the NBA— his own sports fandom—that paved the way for current conversations, starting years ago with his repeated invitations to and visits by colorful and outspoken former Chicago Bulls World Champion Dennis Rodman, the self-proclaimed practitioner of "Basketball Diplomacy" (and also a noted supporter of gay and trans issues). Tigreros said, "If you look at the ancient Olympics, they were held at a time period where no war, no conflict between the city-states would be allowed because they conflicted with the games. The geography of Greece made it impossible for it to be a unified empire, so you had city-states with unique cultures and interests, all armed to the teeth— look at Sparta and Athens. As smart as they were, they realized they needed something to create a cycle of peace, tranquility from a constant state of war. What better way than by having a bunch of athletes representing the different city-states? I think the Olympics have a healing effect, and it's not new."

★ ★ ★ ★ ★ ★ ★ ★ ★ ★ ★

In a nation like China, a new frenzy for the NBA,
international soccer, and global players evade the control
of the Communist elite . . . we regard their contemporary
global presence as antinomian forces that challenge
encrusted sources of domination.
—**Dr. Andrei Markovits, Arthur F. Thurnau Professor,
University of Michigan**

★ ★ ★ ★ ★ ★ ★ ★ ★ ★ ★

A somewhat recent collision of sports with international affairs has been the battle between the NBA and China. A six-word tweet in early October 2019 by Houston Rockets GM Daryl Morey supporting protestors in Hong Kong set this firestorm off. The tweet, which came from Morey's personal account—in no way affiliated with or endorsed by the team or league—repeated the protestors' slogan: "Fight for Freedom, Stand with Hong Kong" and was almost immediately deleted. That's it. Nonetheless, the Chinese government was incensed, canceling television coverage of upcoming NBA games, blocking the sale of Rockets merchandise in China, and demanding Morey's head on a platter, or at least his firing.

The Chinese market has enormous financial value to the NBA—over $4 billion annually according to Victor Cha, author of *Beyond the Final Score: The Politics of Sport in Asia* and a professor and vice dean at Georgetown University, where he recently returned after a three-year sabbatical during which he served on the National Security Council, working on denuclearization negotiations. Cha wrote: "Basketball is the number one sport in China, and there are as many if not more people who play basketball in China than there are Americans in the United States. More than 600 million people in China watched an NBA game in the past season, which is pretty astounding. The emerging Chinese middle-class market for the NBA is larger than the entire population of the United States." China is a big deal for the NBA, but still I found the initial response from the league and players embarrassing and hypocritical. It seemed far more aligned with their economic self-interest than any concerns for either free speech or Hong Kong.

But others, including Michigan professor Andrei Markovits and Cha, sense opportunity for social progress in China via sports fans. At a November 2019 presentation at Georgetown, Cha said:

> While the NBA has said 'we still believe in freedom of expression,' I think both the NBA and agents of the players have basically executed an implicit gag order on players to not say anything about the politics of China. China's leveraging the NBA for

political reasons is very similar in practice to what China has done in other cases. In Norway, when the Nobel Peace Prize Committee gave the Nobel Peace Prize to a Chinese political dissident, China unilaterally stopped the import of Norwegian salmon. They didn't stop salmon from Scotland; they just stopped salmon from Norway. When they got into a dispute with the Philippines, they stopped the import of Filipino bananas. When they got into a dispute with South Korea, they focused on one particular South Korean company and cost them over $2 billion in commercial losses.

So this is a practice we've seen before, but China may have met its match in the NBA, because the big difference is that Chinese people really don't care if they don't eat Norwegian salmon, but they really do care if they can't watch the NBA on TV . . . in this particular issue, China is executing the same sort of strategy they've used in the past but may have bit off more than they can chew.

Sports fandom has clearly not transformed Iran, Iraq, Libya, and Egypt into democratic nations. It has yet to bring free speech to China. At best, in Churchillian terms, soccer was not the beginning of the end for bad governance in these places, but rather the end of the beginning. Yet the bottom line is that passion for sports made things better, and better is much better than nothing.

THE SPORTS FAN AND FAMILY TIES

*D*r. Kristie and her husband have a two-year-old daughter, and she shows me video on her phone of their first attempts to take her out on skis, just at the base of the mountain to get a feel for it, not riding lifts or making turns. As we ride to our last runs of the afternoon, our conversation veers into all things family. I mention how my research has shown that sports spectating has been an important way of spending quality time with family members, and it's also a bond between generations. I recall my own experience with my father, teaching my brother and me how to manually score baseball games in the printed program while we were watching the Mets play at Shea Stadium.

Just about every family that enjoys sports has come together over it. That includes generations of the fanatical Bronco-loving Storey clan. Kelly Storey had bonded as a child with her ailing father over sports, harnessed her passion as a young adult to battle cancer, and later passed on the family traditions to her own daughters, Kasey and Kendra. After she got married, Kelly Storey and her husband bought two Broncos season tickets, even though they had moved to Cheyenne, Wyoming, requiring a three-hour round-trip winter drive for every home game. She attended most games with her husband, but twice a season Kelly would take one of her two daughters for a special mother-daughter bonding experience.

★ ★ ★ ★ ★ ★ ★ ★ ★ ★ ★ ★ ★

We have so many great family stories, memories, moments. I consider myself lucky to have grown up in this family of sports fanatics. It's been awesome growing up Broncos.
—Kasey Storey, as told to the author

★ ★ ★ ★ ★ ★ ★ ★ ★ ★ ★ ★ ★

"We would always get McDonald's on the drive down," Kasey told me. "That's a weird tradition, but those are some of my favorite memories. I remember one game, I must have been ten. It was like thirty-three degrees, cold but just warm enough to rain and not snow, and we were soaked; it's the coldest I've ever been," which is really saying something when you live in Wyoming. "But I made my mother stay the whole game and I told her 'real fans don't leave early.' After it ended we had to go to the fan store and buy all new gear. There are so many moments like that." (They now have ten season tickets, still go to every home game, and make it a family affair with parents, daughters, sons-in-law, and assorted fellow Broncos lovers.)

Watching sports together can also navigate generational age differences, uniting those who might otherwise not have much to talk about. My friend Jim Martel, who works in software in Seattle, went to Boston with his ten-year-old daughter for his father's eightieth birthday, and they all celebrated at a baseball game. Jim and his dad had been going since childhood, and while his father might not understand his career or have much to talk about with a ten-year-old girl, they have baseball. Professor Alan Pringle, who teaches mental health nursing at the University of Nottingham, told the *Huffington Post* that sports give families what he calls a "common currency" connecting them in a way few other activities can, regardless of age or experience: "Most granddads were not that interested in the latest computer games, and most grandsons did not really want to hear what it used to be like to work in a coal mine. But the game offered often three generations of a family a shared experience, shared language, and shared emotion that is not found in too many other areas of life."

My grandmother has a Liverpool Football Club crest on her gravestone. Soccer was the only thing I could talk about sensibly with my father until his death. Eighty percent of my texting and talking with my son is about the team we love. That's a century and counting of [family] history . . . Soccer fandom binds us together in love. It gives us access to a rich, commonly held history that is also intensely personal.
—**Simon Critchley, Hans Jonas Professor of Philosophy, New School for Social Research, in a *New York Times* opinion piece**

When Bill James, the retired editor and publisher of California's *Daily Republic*, a regional newspaper outside of Sacramento, was given tickets to an NFL game from his adult son, the day they shared and all the good memories it brought back moved him so much he wrote a personal essay about it. "My earliest recollections of attending sporting events goes back to the early fifties when the Pacific Coast League still had a franchise in Oakland. My dad would take my brother, Ken, and me to the Oakland Oaks games . . . I was wide-eyed and really didn't know much about the sport, but it was just a kick being at the ballpark with my family."

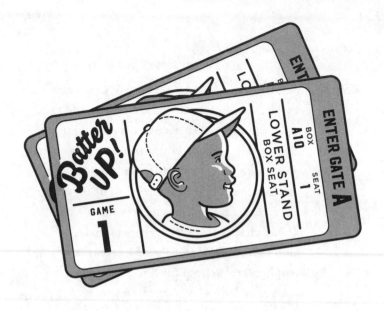

James's family "kick" has run for nearly seventy years, through four generations, and his family's shared love of being together for spectator sports has even helped make the bad memories better. He would attend Dodgers games with his late son, Jeff, who died at age thirty. "I remember the joy on his face when I surprised him one late summer day in 1983. It was his tenth birthday. I had two tickets to the California Angels baseball game and he and I ventured out to celebrate . . . I wish I could once again visit Dodger or Angels stadium with Jeff at my side. But I have those wonderful memories of a shaggy, blond-haired, ten-year-old thrilled to be with dad at a big-league game."

Sometimes the inter-generational bonding of sports fandom plays out in unexpected chronological order. Pulitzer Prize–winning novelist Jennifer Egan considers herself a "reverse second generation" sports fan, one who grew up disinterested and only became captivated with sports after her son did: "Sports are such an absorbing world that I never really knew about much or cared much about until I had a child who was fascinated by all of it. And it's amazing how they provide a kind of structure of meaning in people's lives . . . Things hang in the balance. Outcomes are unclear. There are infinite narratives to it and it's something you can touch in all different areas of your life, at all different times."

Journalist Shankar Vedantam is National Public Radio's social science correspondent and host of the *Hidden Brain* podcast. "You're talking about bonding, and that's clearly a big reason why sports fans are sports fans," said Vedantam on NPR's *Morning Edition*. "We connected with sports teams through family, through our parents taking us to ballgames, and that's why following a sports team feels so intense because it's tied up in these family loyalties." As such, the James gang's story is touching, but hardly unusual. Many families have them. Even, it turns out, Dr. Kristie's.

SPORTS AND OUR BRAINS, PART 3

$\mathcal{A}$s the sun starts to dip lower over the Tetons, we call it a day, stopping at the base of the mountain for an après-ski cocktail and some final thoughts on family traditions in sport. Much to my surprise, our discussion has caused Dr. Kristie to remember some childhood revelations of her own.

"My father used to get tickets to the Bulls, and we would go during those championship years"—her understated way of referring to the half-dozen NBA titles won in back-to-back-to-back three-year championship runs during the Michael Jordan era. She paused and thought about this a bit more before admitting that despite her earlier claim to not be a sports fan, she had "really gotten into it back then." More importantly, she illustrated one of the most surprising psychological aspects of fandom, and one of the reasons why fans, even of losing teams, are usually happier people. The highs are more impactful and memorable than the lows, which quickly fade away, turning a 50–50 season into a winning one in our minds and in turn making us more content than the numbers would suggest. For Dr. Kristie, the great associations of those years, the excitement of Jordan's acrobatic play, and the time spent with her father, all still bring a smile to her face many years later, long after the Bulls dynasty and her interest in spectator sports faded away.

Because "those championship years" she described are widely considered one of the top instances of dominance in the history of sports, Dr. Kristie added a caveat to her just-recalled past happiness: "But that was a special situation."

Except it is not.

In a 2018 essay entitled "Is Fandom Really Worth It?" *Atlantic* contributor and former deputy managing editor Ben Healy begins by noting the obvious: "There's a lot of losing in sports. Only one team can win at a time, and only one champion escapes the season without tears." But then, after diving deeply into the latest research and psychological benefits of fandom, he concludes that "being a fan seems more than anything else to be a matter of managing responses to things one can't control. Sports fans are inclined to respond to reminders of mortality with optimism, and to remember victories much more clearly than defeats. There are surely worse ways to live."

While there are occasional long-running dynasties like the New York Yankees, whose fans have been spoiled by success for decades, and teams that have never won a championship (the NFL's Cardinals infamously claim the longest championship-free history in any major sport at over seventy years), these are anomalies, the extreme highs and lows of team sports. For the vast majority of fans, success falls on the pendulum in between, ups and downs, good years and bad. Over the long term, average teams both win and lose roughly half the time, yet very few fans manage a true zen-master approach, and for the typical sports enthusiast, winning brings emotional joy, sometimes elating, while losing brings sadness, sometimes crushing. You might then think that for most spectators of most sports, the highs and lows should even out, leaving the average sports fan emotionally neutral. But that's not actually the case, because sports fans are built better than that.

It turns out that the highs have almost no limit, especially really big wins like the Cubs' first World Series title in 108 years, a World Cup victory, or pretty much any post-season championship. But if we took losses equally hard, it would be mentally devastating. So, in short, evolution has given the brain an emergency shut off valve to keep things from getting too dire. It is this unconscious circuit breaker that allows almost all sports fans to embrace the thrills of victories more than the agonies of defeat. "You wouldn't go see a movie if you thought there was a fifty-fifty chance you wouldn't like it," says Dr. Daniel Wann, but like many researchers, he believes that sports is simply different from other forms of entertainment. "Sports fans have perfected methods of coping. If they weren't able to cope, there wouldn't be any sports fans."

I want the Cowboys to be the pallbearers at my funeral so they can let me down one last time.
—Dallas Cowboys fan, in the book *Fanaticus*

I suggested the metaphor of a thermostat at your house—set it to sixty-four, and while the temperature may drop, it will never go any lower—and Dr. Wann nodded in agreement that I was following him. In a paper for the *Journal of Sport Behavior* he gets a little more detailed, explaining that while a high level of team identification (fandom) has many measurable mental health benefits: "[H]ighly identified fans are particularly likely to report negative emotion and depression upon witnessing a poor performance by their team. Thus, we are left with a bit of a paradox. How can highly identified persons possess a particularly positive mental health profile if these same persons experience such intense negative responses to their team's losses? . . . the solution to this paradox lies in the defense mechanisms highly identified fans develop to help them cope with their team's poor play and, ultimately, return to a positive mental state ... By employing these defense strategies ... fans are able to (with time) handle their team's failures and once again benefit from the social connections stemming from their allegiance."

In trying to explain the scientific meaning of the "passion" sports fans feel about spectating, Susan Krauss Whitbourne, author of *The Search for Fulfillment* and Professor Emerita of Psychological and Brain Sciences at the University of Massachusetts Amherst surmised, "Obviously, fans are happier when their team wins, but there is also an emotional zeitgeist that develops among spectators that can even override the outcome of the game. The most important of these emotions is that of joy ... You can be entertained, in other words, even if your team loses."

In fact, fans of teams that lose a lot often get an extra boost from the rarity of victories, something social psychologists call "effort justification." Basically, they've put more work into being fans, made more sacrifices along the way, so the good days are that much better. Tufts University psychologist Samuel Sommers and former *Sports Illustrated* executive editor L. Jon Wertheim followed the Mets' surprise appearance in the 2015 World Series, which delighted the Mets' faithful, even though they lost, or more accurately, collapsed. TV announcer Frank Thomas described the outcome this way: "The Mets have nothing to hold their heads down for except they didn't play that well and they gave away this World Series." Nonetheless, the researchers found that among the faithful, "above all there was joy. The fan base . . . was giddy about the season. It wasn't simply that their faith had been rewarded. It was that the previous suffering had imbued the experience with extra sweetness."

It is not uncommon to hear sports fans reminiscing about great moments they enjoyed decades earlier. If your team won just one championship during your lifetime, you probably will remember it, and the joys of success may even grow over time. As leading sports psychology researcher Dr. Rick Grieve told me, "The good times are always better than what they really were."

I was interviewing Ambassador Ronald Weiser about the role of sports fandom in foreign affairs, but because he is a University of Michigan grad and die-hard Wolverines fan, our conversation quickly drifted into college football. He told me, "When your team is successful, you can relive that moment over and over again for years. But you can't relive pain. You are definitely disappointed when your team loses, but then it's in the past. I've been in Ann Arbor when we've won big games. There is a real impact on the fans, they're happier, probably even healthier. It also creates camaraderie and the effect on the community is very powerful. It's a very real thing."

This is one of the most salient conclusions from a new generation of experts studying the sports fan psyche and the myriad benefits of fandom: the pain and disappointment of sports is temporary, while the joy lasts forever.

SPORTS FANS AND VIOLENCE

*W*hen we reconvened in the morning for our final glorious day of skiing, I learned that Dr. Kristie had spent the night considering our earlier discussions: "Last night I got to thinking I should call my dad and chat. I guess I was thinking about our time together at the Bulls' games. It's been a little while and it was so nice. But then I was talking to my husband. You know he's a nurse and he told me he'd heard about a paramedic getting attacked at a baseball game. Isn't that a problem with fans taking these games too seriously? What has your research told you about this issue?"

Yes, violence is a problem, in any almost form; but no, it is not from impassioned fandom. And when it happens at sporting events you definitely hear about it. Unfortunately, that is usually the only time fans make it into the sports pages or onto the evening news. Fortunately, though, it is also extremely rare—so rare that when the media periodically recycles a fan violence story, it typically references incidents that occurred over a decade earlier, because they struggle to find more recent examples. Here is some typical hyperbole: During the 2016 NFL season, after a fight in the stands at a Ravens game, the *Baltimore Sun* ran a story with the headline "Fan brawls are a persistent game-day problem." Then, to prove just how "persistent" they are, in addition to the 2016 incident, the reporter made the obligatory reference back to the days of Roman gladiators, and the equally obligatory reference to Bryan Stow, the most famous American victim of fan-related violence, some five years earlier. Despite mixing multiple professional sports, they managed to come up with exactly one other example in between, for a total of three since 2011. The reporter also cited statistics on stadium arrests at NFL games, without any context, such as noting that these rates are much, much lower than in the world at large. Arrest rates per capita in major American cities routinely run more than 150 times higher than at the stadiums.

But the good doctor's husband was referring specifically to the story of Bryan Stow, a horrible tale that is trotted out by every journalist writing about bad fan behavior both because it is a vivid example of spectators gone bad— though it is dubious whether fandom was even the motivation—and also because incidents like it are thankfully so rare. On baseball's opening day in 2011, Stow, an avid San Francisco Giants fan and paramedic, was beaten nearly to

death by two Dodgers supporters in the Los Angeles stadium parking lot after attending an away game of his team
while dressed in Giants gear. The two assailants, who had
also bothered fellow spectators in the stands during the
game by throwing food and drinking excessively, were sen-
tenced to jail, four and eight years respectively.

Not counting the increasingly long playoff and post-
season games, just the "Big Four" professional sports in
this country drew more than 137 million people in the flesh
to arenas and stadiums in 2017, and except for the (short-
lived) sorrow when their teams lost, the overwhelming
majority went home safe and satisfied.

★ ★ ★ ★ ★ ★ ★ ★ ★ ★ ★ ★

**It gets plenty of publicity when it happens, but sports fan
dysfunction turns out to be remarkably rare.
—Eric Simons, author of *The Secret Lives of Sports Fans***

★ ★ ★ ★ ★ ★ ★ ★ ★ ★ ★ ★

The misperception of fan violence is also exacerbated by
the lingering memories of widespread hooliganism problems in European soccer in the eighties and nineties. While
focused efforts by leagues and governments drastically
reduced that problem in the most prominent organizations
like the Premier League, the bad days still cast a pall over

the image of soccer fans. Fortunately it was never as much of an issue here, and there has been just one game day fatality in more recent US spectator sports memory, when a thirty-year-old Dallas Cowboys fan, now serving twenty years in prison, shot and killed another fan who tried to break up a fight outside AT&T Stadium in 2015. Just one is one too many, but compared to many other things you do outside (or inside) your home, attending sporting events is hardly perilous, and the reality is that the drive to the game is statistically riskier than the game itself.

Dr. Kristie is a charitable soul, so I appealed to that side of her personality. Leaving aside the issues of violence and moving to its opposite, I pivoted. "There's a different aspect of fan behavior that is real, and you might be surprised by it."

"Go on," she said, intrigued.

"Sports fans are more charitable than nonfans."

Higher cash donations and rates of disaster-relief giving, volunteerism, and even giving blood have been documented. In the many charity century bike rides, 10K runs, and walkathons discussed earlier, those who don't turn out to participate often come to volunteer to support those who do. When NFL player J.J. Watt raised nearly $42 million to aid victims after Hurricane Harvey—his goal had been $200,000, half of which he put up himself—*Wall Street Journal* sportswriter Jason Gay told me, "The social media dynamic of fandom is fascinating because it's creating new connections between fans and athletes. Athletes always have had a platform, but now it is more direct between players and their fans. With the J.J. Watt thing, years ago you would have had to drop an envelope in a box at the stadium or mail in a check, now you can give $30 with your phone in a second. Plus, there's Watt tweeting 'We're at $1 million! $4 million! $8 million!' and the fan feels like they are participating." He likened this form of charity to its own kind of competitive sporting event. Dr. Aaron Smith and Dr. Hans Westerbeek, professors at La Trobe University in Melbourne, Australia, studied the effect of sports fandom on volunteerism and charity and concluded that "sport, more than any other potential vehicle, contains qualities that make it a powerful force in effecting positive social contributions."

IT'S JUST A FANTASY

*D*r. Kristie had given some more thought to what we had spoken about the day before. "You talked a lot about the sense of community and the benefits people get from belonging to a tribe, but tribalism can be a bad thing in some ways. Sports fans have always seemed to me to have an 'us versus them' mentality. They love their team but hate other players and other fans. They boo and taunt good players just because they are on another team. That's not good."

I get what she is saying, and to some degree I agree with Dr. Kristie. Comedian Jerry Seinfeld famously questioned this fan-blindness and quipped that we are rooting for laundry, since a team is just players who come and go wearing the same uniforms, and fans only "love" them because of the jersey they wear.

I live in New England, so I know a lot of Red Sox fans, and they tend to "hate" the Yankees more than all the other teams. Part of this is due to proximity, part of it to history as two of the oldest franchises in the game, and no small part of it is envy (the Yankees are arguably the most successful dynasty in any major sport simply in terms of championships and wins), but some of the rivalry goes back to the infamous dealing of up-and-coming prospect Babe Ruth from Boston to New York. It changed sports history and begat Boston's long-running winless streak and "Curse of the Bambino." So Red Sox fans have a special anger for their players leaving the team for pinstripes, which has happened surprisingly often over the years. Outfielder Johnny Damon was an especially beloved Sox star—until he went to the Yankees. Same guy, but hated a day later. A good friend of mine has a rabidly sports-centric college-age (University of Michigan) son (Go Wolverines!) who "loved" Red Sox outfielder Jacoby Ellsbury—until he too went to the Yankees. In both cases the players were branded traitors by Sox fans, and the sports website *BleacherReport* even did an article titled "The 10 Biggest Traitors in Red Sox History," all of them players who had left for the Yankees— even though some were traded against their will, or in the case of Ruth, sold like property.

What exactly was Damon's traitorous act? Taking $3 million more per year than his current team was willing to pay him. Ellsbury's? The Red Sox didn't even offer to renew his contract. Being neither a Yankees nor Red Sox fan, I can be considered an impartial observer and it seems to me that it would be more reasonable for fans to direct their anger at the management of their own team, the ones who refused to pay what the market was willing to bear to keep its beloved hometown stars. But in this respect sports fans are not reasonable, and tribalism takes over. I think Dr. Kristie is right, because feelings like love and hate are too strong to toss around indiscriminately, and it is possible that doing so weakens our understanding of them. Even if it has no real-life repercussions, there is just something ominous to me about team tribalism. But due to a recent paradigm shift, there is now a light at the end of this particular tunnel, and it is getting brighter every season.

★ ★ ★ ★ ★ ★ ★ ★ ★ ★ ★ ★

I fell in love with football as I was later to fall in love with women: suddenly, inexplicably, uncritically, giving no thought to the pain or disruption it would bring with it.
—Nick Hornby, *Fever Pitch*

★ ★ ★ ★ ★ ★ ★ ★ ★ ★ ★ ★

Just like religion, our "choice" of favorite teams usually isn't a choice at all, but rather a fairly arbitrary luck of the draw. Research has shown that far and away the two biggest determining factors of team loyalty (and religion) are where we grow up, and what teams our parents chose.

The most passionate fans I've met—and I've met a lot—
such as those obsessed with the Broncos, Cubs, or Phillies,
though they would be loath to admit (or accept) it, would
almost certainly be equally ardent fans of completely different teams had they simply been born someplace else. Ditto
for college sports, though this is complicated by a third
element—where you went to school. In any case, there is
very little "choice" involved in choosing a favorite team, pro
or college, so yes, in a sense we are all rooting for laundry.
In another sense, we are rooting for our hometown, just
as many people, sports fans or not, are passionate about
where they live or come from.

That being said, whichever team you do end up with,
you still win, and the feeling of being a part of a tribe is
what gives you many of the positive mental health benefits we've seen sports fans enjoy. It is precisely the sense
of group belonging—"us"—that elevates sports fans in
many ways. The "us versus them" rivalry also makes the
competition itself more exciting for most fans, helping produce some of the physiological changes they enjoy during
viewing. But tribalism can also lead to a perceived hatred
toward other teams. For as long as there have been sports,
this has been a dilemma: tribalism and rivalry make our
competitions interesting, but it might be even better if
they didn't threaten our human decency at the same time.
Until recently this has been a minor stumbling block for the

sports fan, but it turns out that maybe we can have it both ways after all.

The big innovation, the "game changer" so to speak, when it comes to fan tribalism, is fantasy sports.

"I'm assuming since you don't watch sports on TV that you have never played fantasy sports?" I asked Dr. Kristie, though I already knew the answer.

In 1961 the Oakland Raiders went a fan-numbing 2–12. Just when it seemed things could not get any worse, the next season began. The Raiders lost their opening game—and then the next twelve—to start a dismal 0–13. In the midst of a depressing late-season East Coast road trip, one of the Raiders owners, Bill Winkenbach, sat in a New York City hotel room with the team's public relations executive Bill Tunnell and *Oakland Tribune* sportswriter Scott Stirling, and in their moment of collective despair, they invented fantasy football, in the form of the Greater Oakland Professional Pigskin Prediction League (GOPPPL).

According to Gary Belsky and Neil Fine, authors of *On the Origins of Sports: The Early History and Original Rules of Everybody's Favorite Games*, GOPPPL was "the first true fantasy sports game and league as we recognize them now . . . Everything a fantasy player today would recognize was present: good humor, bountiful refreshments, obsessive fans, copious rules, and of course, shoddy drafting." As crude as it was—and as few players as there were—the game quickly demonstrated the most important aspect of the future of fantasy sports. When sportswriter Stirling had the very first draft pick in the history of fantasy football, he squandered it and let passion for "his team" overrule common sense, finishing dead last for the season after choosing a hometown hero, Raiders quarterback George Blanda, instead of Jim Brown, whose fifteen touchdowns would propel the team that chose him to GOPPPL's inaugural championship. Ever since then, fantasy sports have been teaching fans a crucially important lesson about tribalism: that the players on "their team," no matter how beloved, are not always the best.

Football was not the first fantasy sport effort—a decade earlier Winkenbach had tried, in vain, to start a fantasy golf league. In 1951, American Professional Baseball Association debuted as the first simulation/strategy sports board game based on real players and their (past) performance, with die rolling and probabilities determining outcomes. Within a decade, it was supplanted by Strat-O-Matic, which until the computer era, become a mainstay in sports-loving households, the baseball fan's version of Monopoly. (It still exists, both as a board game and software version.) I grew up with it and fondly remember endlessly playing Strat-O-Matic baseball with my brother. (The company also rolled out football and hockey versions, but they were never as popular.)

The game my brother and I played was complex, and whether we mixed MLB players all-star style or used actual team rosters, we truly managed our squads, choosing line-ups, deciding when to bunt, steal, put in a reliever, and so on. But while it was based on actual player performance from the previous year, with new cards issued every season, it was still a simulation, a substitute for real spectator sports, something you generally did when not watching a game. The fantasy versions we know today utilize actual player performance in real time and are an extension of, rather than an alternative to, spectator sports, and can be actively participated in while watching TV.

In 1980 Dan Okrent debuted Rotisserie League Baseball, a more complex, realistic, and quickly nationally popular game that could be played without a board or dice, entirely based on real-life, real-time results. In 1984 Bantam Books published the first edition of *Rotisserie League Baseball*, firmly establishing fantasy sports in American culture. While the debut season of GOPPPL, limited to the Raiders' owners' entourage, drew less than ten participants, Rotisserie baseball attracted tens of thousands, and Belsky and Fine describe it as being "rightfully credited as starting the fantasy sports era/craze/movement." The same year, the *1984 Fantasy Football Digest*, a magazine-format publication written by two Minneapolis Vikings fans, debuted, setting out similar real-time rules for America's number-one spectator sport. While it was not initially as well publicized as the Rotisserie book, it lit the fuse that would make football the most popular fantasy option.

While printed rule books lured in more cerebral and devoted sports fans, it was the internet that took fantasy sports mainstream, and the ease of competing on digital platforms caused the popularity to explode exponentially and internationally, eventually becoming the multi-billion-dollar ($7.2 billion in 2017) entertainment business it is today. ESPN put the first serious fantasy football platform online in 1995, the search engine Yahoo introduced free online fantasy play in 1999, and the next big innovation was daily fantasy sports competitions, providing the instant gratification season-long campaigns lacked, such as Fantasy Sports Live and FanDuel.

As the nation's top spectator sport, pro football became the fantasy powerhouse, with 80 percent of those who play virtual sports fielding a virtual NFL team. A special station was even created by the league for fantasy viewers, the NFL RedZone channel, a compilation of all the games going on at once, featuring the highlights of interest to fantasy players. But it's not just football—in the United States there are multiple fantasy leagues for all four major sports, as well as for golf, auto racing, and college football. Overseas, fantasy leagues cater to fans of soccer, cricket, and Australian rules football, among others.

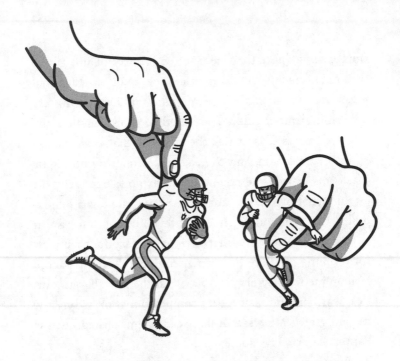

Many of the same benefits we've seen associated with being a fan of real sports—such as increased happiness, larger social networks, multigenerational quality family time, and so on— can also be gained or enhanced though fantasy play. Not surprisingly, given that the more than 59 million North Americans who were regularly participating in fantasy sports in 2017 were already avid sports fans, fantasy sports participants are 57 percent more likely than the general population to belong to a health club or gym. That's to be expected because real-life sports fans exercise more than nonfans. But in terms of societal benefit, fantasy sports breaks new ground in a couple of important ways.

I play because it helps me keep in touch with my friends who I don't see as much anymore. Besides, when I go to school events for my daughter, it gives me something to talk to the other dads about. What else are we going to discuss, politics? No way.
—Tod Minotti, father and fantasy football player, as told to the author

---

Researchers who have looked at motives for fantasy participation have found even greater social and camaraderie aspects than real-life sports. Some have theorized that fantasy sports serve as sort of a social media network all its own, a way for far-flung friends and relatives to keep in regular contact and conversation. In fact, researchers found that the most commonly given motive for playing was "a sense of community and belonging." While sports fans like sports, it seems that fantasy sports fans like one another.

Of course, many fantasy leagues have entry fees and cash prizes, which explains some of the allure. The daily (rather than season-long) internet-based fantasy sites are especially popular with those seeking to profit from their hobby, while in the smaller, social group–based friends and family leagues, the payout is often more of a bragging rights victory, akin to an office March Madness bracket pool or luck of the draw Super Bowl "boxes" lottery.

Temple University professor Joris Drayer and two research colleagues noted that, "Fantasy participants often cite social interaction as one of the primary reasons for their participation. In other words, people like playing fantasy sports because it gives them an opportunity to connect with family, friends, and coworkers . . . These 'communities' are an integral part of the fantasy sport experience." Just as with actually attending games, fantasy can provide a positive family dynamic as a multigenerational activity, but it can do so more frequently and with no concern over cost—unlike going to the stadium. In many households, fantasy sports have taken over the role once held by Scrabble or rummy, a way for children and parents to bond while spending quality time together around the kitchen table, but with even more personal interaction as they plan their draft strategy and analysis. I've talked to a number of parents who "co-manage" teams in partnership with their kids.

As a child, Dan Shepherd would go over box scores with his dad and played baseball simulation games at the kitchen table. Now the avid sports fan and former paratrooper is a father himself: "Sports was a constant source of banter for us around the dinner table growing up, and now it's the same way with me and my son. Yesterday there was a big trade, and that was our dinner conversation." Shepherd has been on the fantasy bandwagon ever since it rolled out on the internet more than twenty years ago. "I started with football back in the nineties and now it's all year round. I love it." He plays in two to four different leagues for each of his three preferred sports (football, baseball, and basketball) sometimes juggling up to a dozen teams a year.

Fantasy sports were a victim of the 2020 coronavirus pandemic, and participants were affected in ways that mainstream sports fans were not. No replays of classic NCAA March Madness tournaments games or even live charity golf events starring Tiger Woods, Phil Mickelson, and Rory McIlroy, along with sports co-stars including Super Bowl champion quarterbacks Tom Brady and Peyton Manning, could provide the stats needed for fantasy to work. "The absence of fantasy sport, I imagine, takes away another coping mechanism during the pandemic," psychologist Cody Havard told me.

But fantasy sports are completely independent of live spectators, and while the return of sports without attendees may have diminished their appeal to traditional fans, and certainly hurt season ticket holders and others who loved to see the games in person, the empty-stadium approach allowed sports to return from the pandemic more quickly, which is all fantasy players needed to fully embrace their passion again. It is also possible that the vast number of Americans introduced to Zoom and other video chatting services and otherwise connecting or reconnecting with friends or relatives they were physically distanced from may discover what fantasy sports players already know: that participation allows them to continue staying socially connected regardless of geography.

Some fantasy sports communities are closer knit than others, and not always by choice. When Gerald Drummond is serving as commissioner of his league, he goes by the moniker Gee Money. It's a brief respite from the other thing he is serving: a life sentence for murder. Drummond is incarcerated in a state prison mental hospital in rural Pennsylvania, as are all the members of his fantasy football league. He started playing after he was released from solitary confinement three years earlier. "This is how we escape our worries for a few hours a week," he told *USA Today* staffers Scott Gleeson and Tom Schad, who wrote, "As fantasy football has become a ubiquitous part of the NFL season, it's also an essential part of prison life. But unlike their counterparts on the outside, prisoners face a unique set of challenges, from staying up on player news with little to no Internet access to keeping track of stats by hand to the potential for violence over gambling and unpaid debts."

The reporters' jailhouse investigation found fantasy sports to be a thoroughly pervasive part of modern prison life all over the country, and while it has obvious appeal in terms of perhaps the most desirable element of any activity in prison—killing time—it also serves higher purposes. Numerous inmates credited the leagues with helping them survive in addition to providing escapism. State University of New York at Fredonia professor Patrick Johnson, who previously worked more than thirty years in the corrections sector and was a prison warden himself, is in favor of staff-monitored fantasy leagues because they can lead to "positive social behavior patterns" and teach prisoners that there's a fun, safe way to spend leisure time when they're released—which 95 percent of all state prisoners will be.

Former San Quentin State Prison chaplain Earl A. Smith is the author of *Death Row Chaplain: Unbelievable True Stories from America's Most Notorious Prison*—and currently the team chaplain for the San Francisco 49ers. He echoed the positive community-building power many traditional sports fans on the outside experience when he told the reporters that, "People who normally wouldn't communicate are friendly with each other. It doesn't matter if a White guy or a Black guy runs the [fantasy] team.

It becomes 'Am I a better evaluator than you?' and 'Can my team beat yours?'" He added, "One of the biggest problems that inmates have when they're released from prison . . . [is] when they have downtime. Teaching them how to spend their leisure time constructively is just as important as teaching them how to work and giving them education programs." When fantasy sports first came on the scene, many real sports leagues opposed it. Why would they not like fantasy sports when it makes viewers watch more games, drives ratings up, funds expanded coverage like the RedZone channel, and profits the leagues' advertisers? Because there is one other big thing fantasy sports does that had those in real sports worried—it creates fans who hate less and like their "enemies" more.

★ ★ ★ ★ ★ ★ ★ ★ ★ ★ ★ ★ ★

I don't think there's any doubt that fantasy sports
has not just increased awareness of the leagues itself,
it's already producing a kinder, gentler sports fan
who can't hate the player on the other team
anymore because he's also on their team.
—*Wall Street Journal* **sportswriter Jason Gay,
as told to the author**

★ ★ ★ ★ ★ ★ ★ ★ ★ ★ ★ ★ ★

"The NFL was initially against fantasy sports, they hated the idea, because they thought it would change the way people viewed sports, that they would stop rooting for teams. But instead, they started watching even more," said psychologist Daniel Wann, who agreed that it has the potential to positively alter the very way the sports fan's mind operates. NCAA President Mark Emmert worries that fantasy sports have the potential to reduce passion at the team level even while bolstering it across the entire sport: "Tribalism can be problematic, but it's also what makes sports great. I like people caring about whether their team wins, and I have concerns about fantasy sports. It can abstract sports—and I have the same problem with gambling. Passion should come from winning, not just covering the spread."

For perhaps the first time in spectator sports, which have been part of **human history** for pretty much all of human history, fantasy sports have forced fans to look beyond their geographic or tribal belief systems and embrace a broader meritocracy that may be rapidly breaking down the longstanding "us versus them" conundrum. It simply becomes much harder to loathe a rival or wish for poor performance by other teams' players when they are now key members of a fan's own fantasy team, and this potentially makes fantasy sports fandom's answer to the familiar question, "Why can't we all get along?"

"For a long time I couldn't draft any players from those 'hated' teams. In my twenty years of fantasy football, as a big Redskins fan, it took me years before I was able to take anyone from the Eagles or Cowboys. But those days are long behind me now," Dan Shepherd told me. "Most definitely it has changed my real-world sports views. I'm a Nats [Washington Nationals] fan, and their big rivals have always been the Phillies and the Braves, but now I have guys from both those teams on my team—and I'm rooting for them in real life."

Shepherd is not the only one. In 2012, a trio of researchers studying fantasy sports among baseball fans concluded that when fantasy players drafted Major Leaguers they had previously disliked, or players from teams they disliked, their disposition toward those players in real life "seriously increased" as a result.

"There's still Notre Dame and Alabama football, there are always going to be these hardcore groups, but the sharp-teeth fan base is going away," the *Wall Street Journal*'s Jason Gay told me, citing fantasy sports as the reason. Kasey Storey's experience affirms this: "My uncle is a Raiders fan, but now I see him rooting for Broncos players, and it's great to see those stalwart rivalries breaking down. It's definitely changed the way I watch football. Now I appreciate all the players—even on teams I once hated. My husband is in a really competitive league and he'd pick his fantasy team over his favorite NFL team."

He's not alone. Research has shown that in just the few short years it has taken fantasy sports to become a big part of American life, they have fundamentally changed the way fans view their allegiances and made their sports worldview more inclusive. Clemson professor John Spinda and psychologist Cody Havard studied the impact of fantasy football on rivalry and determined that, "[W]hile an overall majority of fans . . . preferred a win by their favorite NFL team over a win from their fantasy football team(s), many respondents noted the opposite, preferring a win for their fantasy team over their favorite NFL team." Data shows that some fans now spend more time watching games with their fantasy players on other teams than their own favorite franchise, and the researchers concluded that fantasy participants had fewer negative perceptions about their favorite team's traditional rivals. Other researchers studying fantasy baseball have reached similar conclusions.

Fantasy sports seem to expand benefits already found in sports fandom, such as happiness, self-esteem and bonding, while offering new ones, such as a more benign, less negative attitude toward other teams and their fans. Fantasy is reconnecting far-flung friends and bringing families and co–workers closer together. And that's just for starters, as research into fantasy sports themselves is still in its infancy. University of Houston professor Andrew Baerg studied the way fantasy participants make draft decisions, and what it says about them. Not all fantasy players have let go of tribal favoritism, and not all navigate the complex draft waters of risk, reward, and open-mindedness in player selections, but more are choosing players in a way likely to benefit their fantasy team's performance. "Participation in fantasy sports encourages the expression of what it means to be a productive, well-adjusted citizen in our twenty-first century neoliberal context. As a consequence, fantasy sports participation may have much more far-reaching social and cultural effects than we might imagine," Baerg concluded.

THE UNIVERSAL LANGUAGE

"That's encouraging about fantasy sports and tribalism, and it totally makes sense," said Dr. Kristie. "So do you play?"

"Nope. I never have."

"Why not?"

"I don't really have time for it. You have to follow things pretty closely, watch a lot of games, know the players."

"Don't you already do that?"

"No. I like the NFL and I watch a game now and then, and I sometimes watch post-season baseball, and, of course, *American Ninja Warrior*. But generally I don't spend a lot of time watching sports."

"I thought you were a big sports fan. I thought that was what this book was all about." Dr. Kristie looked really confused.

"I've been in and out of following sports all my life, but never avidly. I've never watched a whole hockey game, and I hardly ever see basketball. What I have become is a fan of sports fans. I find the subject fascinating and game-changing, if you will. For me it's the language of sports that's more important than the games themselves."

"What do you mean?"

Irish poet William Butler Yeats is often credited with the line, "There are no strangers here; only friends you haven't yet met." Several other prominent figures have been similarly linked to it without definitive evidence, but it does sum up a quintessential travel experience, one especially common when visiting the Emerald Isle. I have spent a lot of time in the British Isles, all across England, Wales, Scotland, Ireland, and Northern Ireland, from the big cities of London, Dublin, and Edinburgh to the tip of the Kintyre peninsula, the remote Aran Islands, and many places in between. All of these locales have pubs, and in every one of those pubs, it seems, inevitably, that either cricket or snooker (or both) have been on TV when I've shared a few late-night drinks and good *craic* with the locals. My unwavering ignorance of these sports has always been a successful icebreaker, and at this point, given how many times the finer points of each has been passionately explained to me, you would think I'd be a double-threat snooker/cricket expert by now, but I never seem to remember when I wake up in the morning. This just keeps the phenomenon fresh for me and allows me to meet my next set of newfound friends.

To me what's truly awe-inspiring about sports is this common currency. It erases divides and brings people from all over the world and from every ethnic group and walk of life together. Some of the most ardently passionate sports fanatics I spoke to while researching this book were teenagers, seniors, professors, cab drivers, ambassadors, construction workers, doctors, bartenders, soldiers, students, mayors, governors, and bankers—that is to say they were everyone and anyone, young, old, Black, White, male, female, and so on and so on

Over the last twenty-five years, I have traveled all over the world for work, which means a lot of downtime in airports. All the sizable ones (and most small ones, too) have bars, and every one of those bars has TVs, often lots of them. While one here or there might be tuned to CNN or BBC World News, the rest are almost all devoted to sports, all the time. And you can go into any of those bars in any airport, or pretty much any bar in any city for that matter, and sit down and strike up an enjoyable conversation around sports with a complete stranger from pretty much anywhere. And it doesn't only happen in bars. It happens with your seat neighbor on the plane (or train); you can jump in a cab and chat with the driver; make small talk with shopkeepers; or connect with just about anyone else you interact with.

For example, if you know anything at all about soccer, you have an instant conversation starter with half the world's population, and if you don't, you will almost certainly meet someone wearing a Yankees cap in any corner of the world. You can banter in a way that you can't safely do around religion, or, especially these days, politics, and chatting about weather gets old pretty fast. There is no other oil as effective at greasing the interaction between strangers as sports fandom, period.

★ ★ ★ ★ ★ ★ ★ ★ ★ ★ ★

After many years during which I saw many things, what I know most surely about morality and the duty of man I owe to sport.
—Albert Camus, philosopher, Nobel Prize winner, author of *The Stranger*, soccer fan

★ ★ ★ ★ ★ ★ ★ ★ ★ ★ ★

"Have you ever been in a sports bar?" I asked Dr. Kristie.

"Sure. When I was in college. A few times since then. We don't really have much of that here in Jackson."

"Have you ever thought about the nature of the sports bar and how bizarre it is?" She shook her head. "I mean there are so many other hobbies and forms of entertainment and subjects for discussion, yet there are no opera bars, or weather bars, or movie bars, or politics bars."

But there are sports bars, and there are thousands of them, all around the world. This gathering place appeal of sports consumption is not new, and before Prohibition it was common for fans to gather at saloons near stadiums and listen to baseball games on the radio together—the original sports bar and more evidence of the innate human need for being part of a like-minded group. But the first modern sports bar in the sense of being built as such, Legends, is only forty years young. It was the brilliant idea of retired Los Angeles Rams lineman Dennis Harrah, who went whole hog and stuffed the place with sports memorabilia ranging from a pair of autographed Muhammad Ali boxing gloves to a retired Indy Car hanging from the ceiling. It's the same strategy of souvenir-kitsch-as-props decoration employed by chains Hard Rock Cafe and Planet Hollywood, but those themes are empty—no one actually goes to listen to music or watch movies. At Legends, more than one hundred autographed baseballs are displayed, signed by such greats as Ty Cobb, Babe Ruth, Willie Mays, Joe DiMaggio, and many others, along with endless signed NFL and NBA jerseys, even an autographed pair of Shaq's custom size-23 basketball shoes.

While this kind of stuff is common today, it was unheard of at the time. But the big innovation that made Legends a

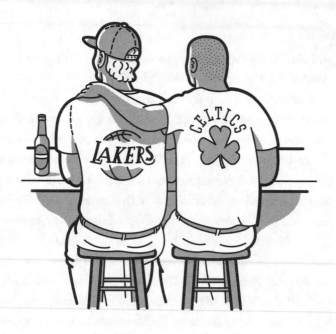

legend, the game changer that spawned a genre of imitators, was being the first bar to leverage the newest technology—satellite television—and broadcast live sporting events from around the world. Legends opened in 1979 in Long Beach, California, and now has a second location in Huntington Beach, and yes, they both serve nachos and chicken wings.

When I am on the road, I'll often pop into a sports bar if I'm by myself, because once you do, you are no longer alone. This is why they are very popular with travelers, as a home away from home where you can go and instantly become part of a community simply by bellying up to the bar, even without being naturally gregarious. Sports bars also function as stadium stand-ins on game day, when fans without tickets want to get dressed up in their logo gear and celebrate with other fans. Many major cities have specific bars that have either positioned themselves as, or evolved into, the known place for expat fans of a particular team to gather and root for their home favorite in "enemy territory." After all, if you are from Wisconsin but your job takes you to the Big Apple, what are you to do? Well, if you googled "Green Bay Packers bar New York" you'd get several hits, including Kettle of Fish, run by a transplanted Wisconsinite. The bar's website states that, "With the exception of Lambeau Field, the Kettle of Fish is the best place to watch a Packers game." New York is so big and has so many transplants that there is a bar for fans of just about every team in every major sport—even for archrival Boston. Professor Thom's in the East Village is decorated with Patriots posters, Tom Brady's college jersey, even original seats from Fenway Park, and it is packed on game nights—whichever Boston team is playing.

The *Huffington Post* ran a story titled "Where to Watch the Dodgers When You're Not in LA," listing fan bars in New York, DC, Boston, and Chicago. What do Broncos-obsessed Denverites do if they move to San Francisco? They go to Nickie's, where one Yelp review reads, "As a Broncos fan in the Bay, this place feels like home for the entire football season." There's even a website, TeamBarFinder.com, that answers such philosophical questions, as what is a Boise State college football fan to do when they find themselves in Portland, Oregon? London's aptly named Jetlag Bar is entirely designed to cater to visiting international fans craving their home team sports (and possibly disoriented by the time change and overnight flight), which are shown on many different flat screens.

But the sports bar is just the most tangible manifestation of the universal language fans share. This commonality also permeates society in many other ways. "During the past two decades my wife and I have taken to the roads of America to see for ourselves the country whose history I have attempted to teach to college students for some fifty years," wrote Richard O. Davies, author of the most widely used college textbook on the subject, *Sports in American Life: A History*. "Everywhere we have traveled in all the fifty states I have been impressed with the pervasive influence of sports . . . Sport in all its many manifestations, transcends time and place and provides a connection for people who have the need to associate with other like-minded individuals . . . As has oft been observed, America is truly a land of many cultures and contrasts. From Miami to Seattle, from Southern California to New England, however, sports provide a common thread, a unifying sense of shared experience, for a nation made up of many and different peoples, cultures, religions, and locales."

History professors Randy Roberts and James Olson studied the impact and importance of spectator sports in American society since World War II: "In a complex society, divided along economic, social, and racial lines, and often sadly impersonal, sports became a currency which all races and classes dealt in. Rich and poor, Black and White, young and old—if they could communicate on no other level, they could always talk about sports."

★ ★ ★ ★ ★ ★ ★ ★ ★ ★ ★ ★

Sport can promote the building of a more fraternal and united world, thus helping to overcome situations of reciprocal misunderstanding between individuals and peoples.
—Pope John Paul II, in a speech

★ ★ ★ ★ ★ ★ ★ ★ ★ ★ ★ ★

Despite the intrinsic tribalism of sports fandom, much of the world is neutral territory, and when you sit down at that airport bar, you don't have to belong to the same team community as your barstool neighbor to erase all these racial, cultural, and professional barriers. You just need to like sports. Or fake it. You'll still be embraced. "When you think of sports fans . . . " wrote science journalist Eric Simons, "fan tribes welcome diversity in a way we often don't."

One of the most interesting descriptions of sports fandom I heard was from baseball historian Mark Langill, who argued that being a sports fan is like having the pass code to a secret society. "You have this alter ego, another identity as a sports fan, and it lets you go anywhere and talk to anyone about things like the standings or managerial strategy."

As University of North Carolina history professor Matthew Andrews explained to me, sounding a bit astonished himself, "They're Republicans, they're Democrats, they have all sorts of different political beliefs. Where else in American society do fifty, eighty, or one hundred thousand people come together for the same event? It doesn't happen anywhere but in sports, except for the biggest multi-day music festivals. In sports you have these weekly scheduled gatherings where so many different people come together."

Maybe we should look to sports fans as role models, instead of the athletes themselves. Yes, at the end of the day, it's just a game, and there are other issues that are more important. But at the same time, fans have no less passion, commitment, or emotion when it comes to their beliefs than people do over politics, yet rival fans can argue and debate incessantly, even angrily, and then immediately return to civility and walk away, still friends. Don't we need this now more than ever?

Overtime

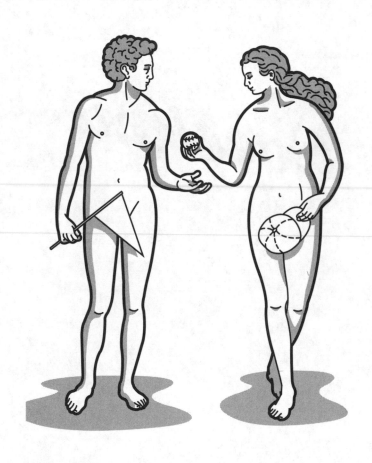

★ ★ ★ ★ ★ ★ ★ ★ ★ ★ ★ ★ ★

"MAN'S JOKE ON GOD"

God says to man, "I've created a universe where it seems like everything matters, where you'll have to grapple with life and death and in the end you'll die anyway, and it won't really matter."

So man says to God, "Oh, yeah? Within your universe we're going to create a sub-universe called sports, one that absolutely doesn't matter, and we'll follow everything that happens in it as if it were life and death."

—Sportswriter Sam Kellerman

★ ★ ★ ★ ★ ★ ★ ★ ★ ★ ★ ★ ★

"Well you've convinced me that the universal language of sports and sports fandom is fascinating because we've been talking nonstop about it for two days, and I'm not even a fan," said Dr. Kristie with a wry smile. "But if, as you said, you're not a big fan, how did you ever come to write this book? Your last one was about food, and I know you love food."

"My father was not a sports fan."

"Huh?"

"When I was growing up my father took my brother and me to baseball games at Shea Stadium. Not all the time, but not infrequently. Before that, he had taken my older sister to see the Brooklyn Dodgers play at Ebbets Field. Sandy Koufax is still her favorite player. After he died, I gave it some thought, and I realized that I never saw him turn on a game on TV. I never saw him read the sports section, and I never saw him show any interest in any other sport. I don't think I ever watched the Super Bowl until college. It dawned on me that he wasn't a sports fan, and I started to wonder about why we'd spent so much time at the ballpark."

The Mets were an expansion team created in 1962 to fill the void left by the twin departures of the city's Dodgers and Giants for greener pastures on the West Coast. My brother and I would join our dad—I don't recall my mother ever attending—in the utilitarian stands, watching America's Game, complete with programs, hot dogs, and all the trappings of the quintessential baseball experience.

My father grew up during the Great Depression and went to work at an early age to help put food on the table. His family took in boarders to get by. When he started college, he rode a single-speed 1940s bike more than two hundred miles because his family had no car, and then, still short of his civil engineering degree, he was drafted into the United States Army Corp of Engineers and shipped off to the Japanese theater. When the war ended, he finished school, joined an international engineering firm, then spent several years building dams in obscure parts of South America. I was not born yet and only know this because years later we loved to watch his home 8mm movies of my dad and his colleagues pushing stuck Land Rovers out of thigh-deep jungle mud.

Faced with serious adult responsibilities from early adolescence to the day he died, my father accomplished a lot of things in his lifetime, but developing a leisure aesthetic was not one of them. A devoted workaholic, he never played golf, bowled, fished, or played cards. He could not even bring himself to truly retire, even in his eighties. When he wasn't working, his sole "hobby" was driving us to designated Historic Civil Engineering Landmarks, those structures that are marked by roadside plaques and ignored by everyone else, then staring in wide wonder at bridge spans or underpasses. In retrospect, he was probably more interested in the stadium itself than what happened there, and may have found the Mets as dull as I found his trestles.

So why did he take us "Out to the Ballgame?" It's a question that never occurred to me as a kid, as a teen, as a college or graduate student, or even during his lifetime. But I've thought about it a lot in recent years, in the greater context of why anyone goes to the game, and why so many make it a family affair. I wish I had asked him when he was alive, but I believe he took us to see the Mets because it was what you did if you wanted to bond with your kids, if you believed family was important even if baseball was not. It would be decades before popular culture coined a term for something my father understood intuitively: quality time.

Dr. Kristie nodded. Even without sports she understands the importance of family and quality time—she is after all a sister, a daughter, a mother, and a wife. Still "not a fan," but now, I think, more understanding of them.

★ ★ ★ ★ ★ ★ ★ ★ ★ ★ ★ ★

[A]t the end of the day, it's just a very pretty game. And it's nice to be around. It's weird—I can't explain it more than that . . . I mean, last October, I traveled to Wrigley Field in Chicago to watch the Cubs lose the sixth and seventh games against the Florida Marlins. And I cared. And I didn't care that I couldn't say why I cared. I just cared. And I still do, and I hope I always will.
    —**George Will, political commentator
    and baseball fan, 2004**

★ ★ ★ ★ ★ ★ ★ ★ ★ ★ ★ ★

Back in 1929, Dr. Abraham Arden Brill, MD, penned what is likely the most famous treatise on sports fandom ever written, *The Why of the Fan*, in which he repeatedly asks the reader "Are you a fan?" Inspired by this, I made it a practice to ask just about everyone I met while researching this book a two-part query, beginning with the similar "Do you consider yourself a sports fan?" If they answered in the affirmative, I immediately asked a follow up: "Do you think being a sports fan has made your life better?" Scores and scores of people, I can't even keep track of how many, from experts I interviewed to friends to strangers in bars, and not one, ever, said no.

One of the most memorable answers came from Las Vegas Mayor Carolyn Goodman, under whose tenure what had been the biggest city in the nation without a pro sports team in one of the four major sports suddenly got two, NHL hockey and NFL football. "Without a doubt. I am an enormous sports fan, and yes it has definitely affected my life for the better. The whole world of sports is such a learning experience for every human being if they take the time out to appreciate it, it can give you so much. Sport is a magnificent piece of life."

While we may come to sports with stereotypes or preconceptions, as I did, and Dr. Kristie did, sports fandom is not highbrow or lowbrow, it's everywhere and among every group of people. It's part of life, and like the meaning of life itself, it may remain inexplicable. Yet while the reasons for our widespread love of sports may be enigmatic, with all these subtexts and deeper meanings and higher purposes rolled up into it, there is one aspect of the mystery I think I have solved. I'm now sure that it's a good thing, a very fine thing, to be a fan. It's also a lot of fun.

ACKNOWLEDGMENTS

"There is no 'I' in TEAM"

—Anonymous

Over and over again in the past few years I heard about how much power sports has to bring people together, and I found that to be especially true when it came to getting people to talk to me. As a journalist for well over twenty years, I've interviewed a lot of people, and I've also not interviewed a lot of people, because they've refused. However, this time, virtually no one I really wanted to talk to turned me down. I found that sports was a key that opened even the most securely locked doors, and almost without exception, people were willing to spend their valuable time talking to me about sports, often in conversations that sprawled longer and broader than I had promised them. Why? Because people love to talk sports. In many cases they literally can't help themselves. From nationally prominent politicians to leaders of large organizations who rarely give interviews to people who had suffered some horrible incident that they could only discuss through tears, I was surprised and remain profoundly thankful how willing and eager people were to open up to me and talk sports. Beyond that, some welcomed me into their lives, their offices, bought me drinks, met me for coffee, and much more.

Also, believe it or not, entire lengthy sections of this book ended up being cut. As a result, many of the highest profile and most interesting people I spoke to, will not find their names in the preceding pages, but they took the time to speak to me nonetheless, and I thank them for that. This subset includes mayors, governors, CEOs, professional athletes, friends, a team mascot or two, and a potential future president of the United States. Most of all, it pained me to lose the many hopeless romantic sports enthusiasts I spoke with who met, got engaged, or even were married at or in conjunction with major sporting events.

So the list of those I'm thanking is long, but some of the many people who were invaluable in writing this book includes world class sports fan researcher Dr. Daniel Wann, his colleagues Dr. Rick Grieve and Dr. Cody Havard, and all the experts who attended their annual psychology conference and shared insights and the newest research data with me. From the realm of social and political studies, I thank political science professor Andrea Talentino, and all the experts who attended her interdisciplinary sports conference and similarly shared their ideas with me. For their insights into diplomacy, geopolitics, and the joys of being Cubs and Wolverines fans respectively, I thank Ambassador Peter DeShazo and Ambassador Ronald Weiser, along with US Navy vet Carlos Tigreros, who sat out his embassy's World Cup viewing parties in protest of Putin's policies and made me rethink the role of unlikely global peace ambassador Dennis Rodman—Carlos, thank you for your service.

In Indiana, a living, breathing laboratory of the benefits of sports fandom, an extra special five-star VIP thanks to Chris Gahl, Butler trustee and the unofficial mayor of Indianapolis; real-life former Indy Mayor Greg Ballard; Indiana Governor Eric Holcomb; Indiana sports development legend, philanthropist, United Nations official, and public servant James Morris; former Indy 500 and Indianapolis Motor Speedway boss Mark Miles; Indiana Sports Corp President Ryan Vaughn; USA Football President Scott Hallenbeck; Colts Vice President Steve Campbell; Trey Mock, aka "Blue"; Pacers announcer and former Butler Athletic Director Chris Denari; WNBA legend Tamika Catchings; local son Pete Dye, the most awarded golf course architect in history; WTHR cameraman Rusty Hornickel; WTHR news anchor Carlos Diaz; Hoosier legend Bobby Plump, who makes the best pork tenderloin sandwich in a city famous for them; all the folks at legendary steakhouse

St. Elmo's, my favorite sports-related dining spot in the world; and especially NCAA President Mark Emmert, who was gracious, forthcoming, and very knowledgeable.

In Las Vegas, Mayor Carolyn Goodman; Golden Knights SVP Brian Killingsworth; unofficial mayor Scott Ghertner (whom even my Uber driver knew—everyone does), the most avid sports fan I know who has not taken the plunge into costumed "superfandom"; UNLV Associate Men's Hockey Head Coach and shooting survivor Nick Robone; and Jessica Duran, who most definitely did not have to talk with me but did anyway, and was awesome. And to all the Golden Knights fans I spoke to, bartenders, taxi drivers, and pretty much everyone in Vegas, more thanks. Go Knights! (I have never been a hockey fan, and I have especially not been a fan of wearing logo gear. But as I left the Knights' executive office on my last day in Vegas doing interviews, I did something I have not done in well over a decade—I walked into the gift shop and bought a Knights hat. It felt like a community worth being part of, even very peripherally, and was much easier than getting inked.)

In Colorado, state ambassador par excellence Carly Holbrook; former governor, former Denver mayor and craft beer guru John Hickenlooper; Taylor Shields, who knew so much about so many different areas of sports fandom simply by being a fan; Allie Pisching and Seth Medvin at the

Denver Broncos; and Rich Grant, whose lifelong dream of legal marijuana finally came true.

In Detroit, another very special extra VIP thanks to close friend, award-winning broadcaster, newspaper journalist, and prolific author Michael Patrick Shiels, host of the state's number-one drive time radio talk show, *Michigan's Big Show*—tune in now! (You can listen on internet radio anywhere in the world.) Besides invaluable perspective on the Motor City Miracle, Shiels was a fountain of connections and suggestions, and for years has put smiles on my face and golf trophies on my shelves through our never-ending global match.

In Wyoming, the inspirational Kelly Storey, who I hope to one day take in a Broncos game with.

My Hoya friends from Georgetown, sports fans one and all: John Bonina, Joe Kresse, Jim McGrail, Bob Stein, Joe LaPlante, Pete Clare, Joe Feeney, Soumi Eachempati, Jeff Bradley, Takeski Kawamoto, all the others I'm forgetting, and the late Peter Murphy—thank you for your service.

Thanks to all my other sports-mad friends who gave me perspective, too numerous to list here, but especially Dan Shepherd (thank you for your service), Jacob Peress (Go Wolverines!), Art Keating, and Liz DeLucia, who once drove the Zamboni at Boston Garden. Special thanks to my inner circle of friends that I have actually traveled with to attend great events in person, Robert Pedrero, Jim Martel, Pat Gallagher, and my wife, who certainly would not have ever gone to a car race—actually two of them—otherwise. To my late father, who took me to so many Mets game growing up, my brother who was a frequent ballpark companion, and my sister, who has thrown awesome launch parties for my last two books, and who will undoubtedly step up to the plate and once again knock it out of the park (and as an aside, had Yankees season tickets for eight seasons, some 648 home games, and took my wife as her guest, once—just saying).

Kate Monaghan and Hicks Wogan at the 9/11 Memorial Museum in New York City (go—it is awe-inspiring, and was just rated the nation's number-one museum).

Wall Street Journal sportswriter and social pundit Jason Gay whose only sportive failing is retweeting the lame BikeSnobNYC way too often; Los Angeles Dodgers team historian Mark Langhill; Kenneth Shropshire, author, attorney, professor, and CEO of the Global Sports Institute at Arizona State University; religion expert/Ivy League professor/priest/Detroit Lions fan Dr. Randall Balmer; Andrew Zimbalist, the Robert Woods Professor of Economics at Smith College; Professor Matthew Andrews, obsessed with sports at UNC; Professor Alan Castel at UCLA; mega-best-selling author Mark Bowden, whose non-sports books *Blackhawk Down*, *Killing Pablo*, and *Guests of the Ayatollah* kept distracting me from doing actual work and who is an extremely generous person; the Nashville Predators, Indiana Pacers, and other pro and college teams I am sure I'm forgetting.

To the Buffalo Bills—New York state's only professional football team—who taught me the hard way that winning is not everything and that you can still enjoy being a fan even in the face of historically anomalous and statically highly improbably back-to-back-to-back-to-back Super Bowl losses.

For insights into South Africa, golf legend Gary Player, who was so gracious and giving in our one-on-one chat; the indominable Alan Petersen, arguably the world's most famous safari guide (call Micato Safaris), and whose services are the only thing I have in common with people like Warren Buffet and Hillary Clinton when it comes to the style I travel in; and former sportscaster-turned-travel-agent-to-the-stars Chad Clark (if you ever want to attend the Super Bowl, Kentucky Derby, Masters, or other "bucket list" sports event, just contact Chad Clark Travel in Phoenix, Arizona).

Wishing long love and many games together to fan couples Austin and Taylor Klein and Morgan and Conor Payne.

To some of the relatively few, but still mighty, authors who stuck their toe into the murky waters of the importance of sports fandom and deeply influenced me, including

Franklin Foer (*How Soccer Explains the World*), Warren St. John (*Rammer Jammer Yellow Hammer*), John Carlin (*Playing the Enemy*), Eric Simons (*The Secret Lives of Sports Fans*), and Mark Frost (*The Greatest Game Ever Played*).

Another extra special thank you to Dr. Doug Scothorn, Buddy, Kyle, Jamie Sandys, and all the wonderful folks at the Make-A-Wish Foundation, an incredibly worthy organization that moved me emotionally (and is worthy of a donation).

A penultimate extra special thanks to the real-life Dr. K, who never had the slightest idea that our background conversation during a fun day of skiing, years into my research, inspired me to rethink my entire concept in terms of a Socratic conversation with a non-sports fan. When you are on the inside of a topic, it's easy to get wrapped up in all you think you know about it, and her blissful ignorance of all things sports fan-esque (expect the Michael Jordan–era Bulls) enlightened me with her perspective. You ask questions in order to learn things, but in this case, I learned more from the questions she asked.

A final extra special thanks to my very capable research assistant, skilled writer, and resolutely self-aware sports fan Kasey Storey.

To all the folks at Algonquin Books, where my previous book was such a good experience (not the norm) that I really wanted to keep the team together for this one. Alas, we lost an MVP or two to free agency, but I'm still hopeful about our chances.

To Zarafa, my four-legged personal trainer, who forced me to go for walks and hikes when I was otherwise housebound and obsessed with obsessed sports fans, then spent countless hours sitting under my desk while I typed these words. Many moments of clarity, breakthroughs, and editorial resolution came while in the woods, safely off-line.

Last but certainly not least, my wife, Allison, who proofed chapters in a series of late-night frenzies, picked a huge upset winner in the Kentucky Derby, and occasionally pretends to be interested in *American Ninja Warrior*. As I write this, her Yankees are—surprise, surprise—once again playing in the post-season.

END GAME

Pre-Game

Forty thousand pilgrims would assemble; C.L.R. James, *Beyond a Boundary*, (London: Stanley Paul & Co., 1963; Chapel Hill: Duke University Press reprint, 2013), 155.

Game Time

"[A]re you a fan? A. A. Brill, *The North American Review*, Vol. 228, No. 4 (Oct. 1929), 429-434.

Scott Simon, the NPR Weekend Edition Saturday host Scott Simon, *Home and Away: Memoir of a Fan*, Hyperion, New York, 2001, 12

Longtime ESPN television producer Justine Gubar, *Fanaticus*, Rowman & Littlefield, Lanham, MD, 2015, 139

Are sports fans lazy? Wann, Daniel L., Merrill J. Melnik, Dale G. Pease, Gordon W. Russell, *Sports Fans: The Psychology and Social Impact of Spectators*, (New York: Routledge, 2001), 157.

Sports Fans Are Happier People

The purpose of our lives Wallace J. Nichols, *Blue Mind: The Surprising Science That Shows How Being Near, In, On, or Under Water Can Make You Happier, Healthier, More Connected and Better at What You Do*, (New York: Little Brown & Co., 2014), 16.

People's lives are enriched https://www.wkms.org/post/murray-state-present-abcs-sport-fandom-what-we-know-and-where-we-should-go#stream/0

He jokes that when he began studying Ibid.

In his three-plus decades of research Wann, D. L., & Martin, J. (2008). "The positive relationship between sport team identification and social psychological well-being: Identification with favorite teams versus local teams." *Journal of Contemporary Athletics, 3,* 81-91.

more vigor and less fatigue Wann, D. L., & Weaver, S. (2009). "Understanding the relationship between sport team identification and dimensions of social well-being." *North American Journal of Psychology, 11,* 219-230.

Some of the biggest pluses Wann, D.L (June 2007) *North American Journal of Psychology* 9.2, 251.

What we call the ABCs https://www.wkms.org/post/murray-state-present-abcs-sport-fandom-what-we-know-and-where-we-should-go#stream/0 (audio portion)

But it can also provide a sense Ibid.

A feeling of belonging http://www.nytimes.com/2000/08/11/sports/sports-psychology-it-isn-t-just-a-game-clues-to-avid-rooting.html?_r=0

"The benefits of social support Wann, D. L. (2006) *Journal of Sport Behavior* Examining the potential causal relationship between sport team identification and psychological well-being, *29,* p.80.

Nearly eighty million living https://www.forbes.com/sites/stuartanderson/2018/04/27/27-of-major-league-baseball-players-are-foreign-born/#483a836e7712

A joint global project Doyle, Jason, Kevin Filo, Daniel Lock, Daniel C. Funk, and Heath McDonald, "Exploring PERMA in spectator sport: Applying positive psychology to examine the individual-level benefits of sport consumption," *Sport Management Review,* 19.5, November 2016, 506–519.

"Humans are inherently tribal creatures Leon Neyfakh, *Boston Globe*, How Teams Take Over Your Mind, April 24, 2011 p. K4

"For tens of millions of Americans, Roberts, Randy and James Olson, *Winning is the Only Thing: Sports in America since 1945,* Johns Hopkins University Press, Baltimore, 1989, xii

In 2018, these included Sunday Night Football https://bestlifeonline.com/most-watched-tv-moments-2018/

More than decade ago Wann, D. L. (2006). "Examining the potential causal relationship between sport team identification and psychological well-being." *Journal of Sport Behavior, 29,* 79-95.

Researchers Chaeyoon Lim https://www.pewforum.org/2019/01/31/religions-relationship-to-happiness-civic-engagement-and-health-around-the-world/

Karolina Krysinska and Karl Wann, D. L., Waddill, P. J., Brasher, M., & Ladd, "Examining sport team identification, social connections, and social well-being among high school students," *Journal of Amateur Sport*, *1*(2), 2015, 28.

Wann and his colleagues looked into Ibid.

If you are lonely https://appliedsportpsych.org/site/assets/documents/FanBehaviorcanimpactathletes.pdf

Sports as Entertainment

A 2017 study by researchers Jenna Birch, *Washington Post*, "How Binge-watching is hazardous to your health," June 3, 2019. https://www.washingtonpost.com/lifestyle/wellness/how-binge-watching-is-hazardous-to-your-health/2019/05/31/03b0d70a-8220-11e9-bce7-40b4105f7ca0_story.html?noredirect=on&utm_term=.2b07d70d3dd4

In a Washington Post feature Ibid

"Sports fans are not just simply sitting https://www.wkms.org/post/murray-state-present-abcs-sport-fandom-what-we-know-and-where-we-should-ga#stream/0

"I believe and hope to prove C.L.R. James, *Beyond a Boundary*, (London: Stanley Paul & Co., 1963; Chapel Hill: Duke University Press reprint, 2013), 154-5.

"[T]here is one crucial dimension Andrei S. Markovits & Lars Rensmann, *Gaming the World*, Princeton University Press, Princeton & Oxford, 2010, 47

Mark Bowden, the author Mark Bowden, *The Best Game Ever*, Atlantic Monthly Press, New York, 2008, 195

Sports and Our Brains

Dr. Alan Castel https://www.psychologytoday.com/us/blog/metacognition-and-the-mind/201310/can-following-baseball-be-good-your-brain

A 2008 study by University https://www.prevention.com/life/a20436977/health-benefits-of-being-a-sports-fan/

Sian Beilock, an associate psychology https://www.cnn.com/2012/04/13/health/side-effects-sports-fan/index.html

Journalist Lizette Borelli pursued https://www.medicaldaily.com/mind-and-body-sports-fan-sports-games-388444

*But that is no*t the typical fan, Wann, D. L. (2006). "Examining the potential causal relationship between sport team identification and psychological well-being." *Journal of Sport Behavior, 29,* 79-95.

Despite the fact Warren St. John, *Rammer Jammer Yellow Hammer*, Crown Publishers, New York, 2004, 130-1

Well, college students Eric Simons, *The Secret Life of Sports Fans: The Science Of Sports Obsession*, Overlook Press, NY, 2013, 205

Most notably, she held up https://www.cnbc.com/2018/04/27/7-sports-strategies-you-can-use-to-succeed-in-business.html

Sports and Our Brains, Part 2

Australian doctors inserted http://www.dailymail.co.uk/health/article-2513232/Even-just-WATCHING-sport-improve-fitness.html

This is how cognitive scientist Sian https://news.uchicago.edu/story/athletes-and-spectators-brains-light-when-talking-sports

At the Spaienza University of Rome Eric Simons, *The Secret Life of Sports Fans: The Science Of Sports Obsession*, (New York: Overlook Press, 2013), 71.

To test levels of testosterone http://nautil.us/issue/39/sport/the-unique-neurology-of-the-sports-fans-brain

A researcher in Lisbon did Eric Simons, *The Secret Life of Sports Fans: The Science Of Sports Obsession*, (New York: Overlook Press, 2013), 22-23.

In a similar vein, Robin Dando https://www.abcactionnews.com/lifestyle/food-tastes-better-and-other-side-effects-when-your-team-is-winning-the-game

In Blue Mind, *his water* Wallace J. Nichols, Blue Mind, Little Brown & Co., New York, 2014, p. 259-60

A Houston Aeros hockey fan Wann, Grieve, Zapalac, End, Lanter, Pease, Fellows, Oliver, and Wallace (2010). "Examining the superstitions of sports fans: types of superstitions, perceptions of impact, and relationships with team identification." *Athletic Insight Volume 5, Number 1*

Wann and eight colleagues, representing Wann, Grieve, Zapalac, End, Lanter, Pease, Fellows, Oliver, and Wallace (2010). "Examining the superstitions of sports fans: types of superstitions, perceptions of impact, and relationships with team identification." *Athletic Insight Volume 5, Number 1*

Post-Traumatic Recovery: How Sports Heals Communities

Psychologists and professors Yuhei Inoue Inoue, Yuhei & Havard, Cody, "Sport and disaster relief: a content analysis," *Disaster Prevention and Management*, 2015, Vol. 24 Issue 3, 355—368.

"In just one year, 2013 Inoue, Yuhei & Havard, Cody, "Sport and disaster relief: a content analysis," *Disaster Prevention and Management*, 2015, Vol. 24 Issue 3, 355—368.

Tonight there will be "Comeback Season: Sport After 9/11" 2018 special exhibition at 9/11 Memorial Museum, New York City.

"Walking through the museum https://www.huffingtonpost.com/wicked-good-travel-tips/911-tribute-walking-tour-_b_1770647.html

The opening review https://nypost.com/2014/05/15/new-911-museum-is-as-beautiful-as-it-is-horrific/

What people look for in sports Paul Newberry, *Associated Press*, "It's Time for Sports to Help Us Heal Again," April 20, 2013

Sport to given as our sense Ibid.

After the game, Piazza https://nypost.com/2016/07/18/how-sept-21-2001-unfurled-at-shea-when-piazza-made-ny-smile/

Howie Rose, the Mets Ibid.

Years later, after retiring https://www.si.com/mlb/2016/09/21/chipper-jones-braves-mets-mike-piazza-home-run-september-11-attack

"Going to the game was very difficult http://www.nydailynews.com/sports/baseball/mets/9-11-family-forget-mets-piazza-article-1.1470645

When that ball went over the wall "Comeback Season: Sport After 9/11" 2018 special exhibition at 9/11 Memorial Museum, New York City.

After the game http://www.nydailynews.com/sports/baseball/mets/9-11-family-forget-mets-piazza-article-1.1470645

Whatever you call it https://en.wikipedia.org/wiki/2017_Las_Vegas_shooting

"It's as improbable as CBS This Morning, Saturday Edition, June 2, 2018

"We wanted to win Ibid.

As with 9/11, it began https://theathletic.com/314477/2018/04/15/britton-how-the-red-sox-helped-heal-boston-in-wake-of-the-marathon-attack/

Red Sox catcher David Ross Ibid.

Sports and Spiritual Healing

In 2017, on the fiftieth https://www.theoaklandpress.com/sports/pat-caputo---years-later-riots-and-tigers-define/article_90b5f4d7-92d2-5616-9687-66d7ac179689.html

Former New York Times https://wdet.org/posts/2017/07/28/85557-how-significant-was-the-1968-world-series-after-the-1967-uprising/

On the night before http://www.staradvertiser.com/2018/08/24/breaking-news/little-league-world-series-honolulu-team-send-their-aloha-to-hurricane-weary-hawaii-in-video/

CBS Sports *wrote* https://www.cbssports.com/general/news/little-league-world-series-as-hurricane-lane-approaches-hawaii-is-playing-for-more-than-a-trophy/

Hawaii won Ibid.

"My ex-husband ran away https://www.nytimes.com/2018/07/05/obituaries/michelle-musler-courtside-perennial-in-the-garden-dies-at-81.html

Sports Heals

There have been so many that https://www.milehighreport.com/2016/10/9/13215660/denver-broncos-hard-won-path-to-super-bowl-50-paralleled-a-battle-against-cancer

Science writer Eric Simons Eric Simons, *The Secret Life of Sports Fans: The Science Of Sports Obsession*, (New York: Overlook Press, 2013), 144.

The most recently completed such study Shoshani, A. Mifano, K. Czamanski-Cohen, J. (2015). "The effects of the [Make-A-Wish] intervention on psychiatric symptoms and health-related quality of life of children with cancer: a randomized controlled trial." *Quality of Life Research,* 25(5), 1209-1218. doi 10.1007/s11136-015-1148-7

When the hospital built George Schroeder, *USA Today*, "Iowa Wave Through the Eyes of a Child," November 3, 2017, C1

It started when Iowa football Ibid

On video, it's a simple yet Ibid

The idea immediately went viral Ibid

Building A Better Sports Fan

In 2012 a group of researchers L.Gregory Appelbaum, Matthew S.Cain, Elise F.Darling, Steven J.Stanton, Mai Thi Nguyen and Stephen R. Mitroffac, *Personality and Individual Differences*, Volume 52, Issue 7, May 2012, p. 862

I had got into the Olympic https://olympiclegacynews.wordpress.com/2012/11/18/hello-world/

In one study, the Sporting https://www.sfia.org/press/431_SGMA-Says-The-Olympics-Do-Impact-Sports-Participation

According to research by the International https://serval.unil.ch/resource/serval:BIB_945142D46802.P001/REF p.101

After Beijing, researchers found https://www.sfia.org/press/431_SGMA-Says-The-Olympics-Do-Impact-Sports-Participation

While some people may not be Ibid.

"What's really exciting for us https://www.clubindustry.com/profits/24-hour-fitness-sees-membership-increase-olympic-exposure

After the 2000 Sydney Olympics https://serval.unil.ch/resource/serval:BIB_945142D46802.P001/REF p98

while Britain saw a respectable http://www.bbc.com/future/story/20160805-do-big-sporting-events-make-us-do-more-sport

The 1992 Barcelona Games https://serval.unil.ch/resource/serval:BIB_945142D46802.P001/REF p.95

But another Canadian study found http://www.bbc.com/future/story/20160805-do-big-sporting-events-make-us-do-more-sport

"Somewhat improbably, even as the house https://www.denverpost.com/2013/03/28/lance-armstrong-launched-a-generation-of-bicyclists/

According to Canada's CBC News https://www.cbc.ca/news/world/how-lance-armstrong-transformed-north-american-culture-1.1234593

According to Prevention, https://www.prevention.com/life/a20436977/health-benefits-of-being-a-sports-fan/

Using cutting edge http://www.dailymail.co.uk/health/article-2513232/Even-just-WATCHING-sport-improve-fitness.html

One of the researchers Ibid.

According to Dr. Wann Daniel L. Wann, Merrill J. Melnik, Gordon W. Russell, Dale G. Pease, *Sports Fans: The Psychology and Social Impact of Spectators*, (New York: Routledge, 2001), 157.

His studies have variously https://www.prevention.com/life/a20436977/health-benefits-of-being-a-sports-fan/

"The march of the American women Richard O. Davies, *Sports In American Life (A History)*, 3rd Ed., 2017, John Wiley and Sons, Malden, MA, 381

Ninety-two thousand fans Ibid., 382

"Very few, if any, American Andrei S. Markovits & Lars Rensmann, Gaming The World, Princeton University Press, Princeton & Oxford, 2010, 202

It was a watershed moment Richard O. Davies, Sports In American Life (A History), 3rd Ed., 2017, John Wiley and Sons, Malden, MA, 384

After twenty-year old Francis Ouimet Ibid., 144-5.

When Jones arrived Ibid.

three-quarters of the courses https://www.ngf.org/golf-industry-research/

median peak-season https://golftips.golfweek.com/average-cost-round-golf-20670.html

Twenty-First Century Sports Fans: *American Ninja Warrior*

In the summer of 2018, https://www.thewrap.com/american-ninja-warrior-bachelorette-men-tell-all-ratings/

American Ninja Warrior pulled in https://ew.com/tv/2017/12/19/75-most-watched-tv-shows-2017-18-season/

By mid-2018 there were https://globalsportmatters.com/business/2018/08/17/popularity-tv-show-spurs-growth-ninja-training-gyms/

Less than a year later https://www.ninjaguide.com/anw-ninja-warrior-training-gyms/usa/

"People are looking for some way https://globalsportmatters.com/business/2018/08/17/popularity-tv-show-spurs-growth-ninja-training-gyms/

Steve Kimpton, instructor https://www.azcentral.com/story/news/local/scottsdale/2018/09/01/american-ninja-warrior-leads-growth-ninja-training-gyms/1135260002/

"Inspired by the television series http://www.baltimoresun.com/features/bs-fe-ninja-warrior-workouts-20170609-story.html

We aspire to become what we see https://www.americanninjawarriornation.com/2016/8/23/12619194/american-ninja-warrior-gyms-workouts-leading-fitness-revolution

Wall Street Journal *sportswriter Jason Gay* https://www.wsj.com/articles/is-american-ninja-warrior-the-future-of-sports-1464707294

Bad Fans or Bad Role Models?

after serving jail time http://www.nfl.com/news/story/09000d5d801c20fc/article/timeline-of-michael-vick-dogfighting-case

And the hordes of fans https://en.wikipedia.org/wiki/Philadelphia_Eagles

In the past decade, several dozen http://harvardjsel.com/2015/07/bethany-withers-without-consequence/

and the idea that the Atlantic https://www.theatlantic.com/notes/2016/09/nfl-concussions/499841/

In the first full regular season https://www.usatoday.com/story/sports/nfl/2019/01/24/nfl-says-concussions-down-29-percent-in-regular-season/38949807/

and that the conclusion of his guilt https://en.wikipedia.org/wiki/Deflategate

One of the best-known examples https://www.sbnation.com/nfl/2014/5/23/5744964/ray-rice-arrest-assault-statement-apology-ravens

NFL Commissioner Roger Goodell Ibid.

(In a 2010 incident https://www.vice.com/en_us/article/bmwe8w/ben-roethlisberger-quarterback-twice-accused-of-sexual-assault

A year before the nightclub incident Ibid.

As spring training for baseball's 2019 https://chicago.suntimes.com/sports/cubs-addison-russell-returns-spring-training-braces-fans-wrath-domestic-violence-suspension/

Sports Fans and Civil Rights

As Michigan Professor Andrei S. Markovits and Steven L. Hellerman, *Offside: Soccer & American Exceptionalism*, 2001, Princeton University Press, Princeton NJ, 131.

America lived and breathed Ibid., 68.

Robinson's entire baseball career Joseph Dorinson and Joram Warmund, Ed., Jackie Robinson: Race, Sports and the American Dream, M.E. Sharpe, Armonk, NY, 1999, 208.

"Barack Obama would never have https://www.huffpost.com/entry/ken-burns-explain-why-the_b_9655134

After all, so does Obama https://www.chicagotribune.com/sports/cubs/ct-obama-sports-cubs-white-house-spt-0117-20170116-story.html

Reverend King himself: https://kinginstitute.stanford.edu/encyclopedia/robinson-jackie

The coauthors of Patrick Miller & David Wiggins, Ed., *Sport and The Color Line*, Routledge, 2004, New York, 173.

New York sportswriter Lester Rodney Dave Zirin, *What's My Name Fool, Sports and Resistance in the United States*, Haymarket Books, Chicago, 2005, 33.

Sometimes it's not enough to change https://www.chicagotribune.com/sports/cubs/ct-obama-sports-cubs-white-house-spt-0117-20170116-story.html

Consider this: a 2017 study https://www.fotball.no/globalassets/dommer/the-future-sports-fan_spilleregler_english.pdf

I put the obvious question to Cole Warren St, John, *Rammer Jammer Yellow Hammer*, New York: Crown Publishers, 2004), 216-7.

In The Boys of Summer, Patrick Miller & David Wiggins, Ed., *Sport & The Color Line*, Routledge, 2004, New York, ix.

"Minimal group theory" is an, Sally Kohn, *The Opposite of Hate*, Algonquin, 2018 Chapel Hill, 104.

Or as science writer Eric Simons, *The Secret Life of Sports Fans: The Science Of Sports Obsession*, (New York: Overlook Press, 2013), 220-1.

After his death, Robinson's wife Joseph Dorinson and Joram Warmund, Ed., *Jackie Robinson: Race, Sports and the American Dream*, M.E. Sharpe, Armonk, NY, 1999, 212.

In his first season Patrick Miller & David Wiggins, Ed., *Sport & The Color Line*, Routledge, 2004, New York, 185.

By the end of that very first Richard O. Davies, *Sports In American Life (A History)*, (Malden, MA: John Wiley and Sons, 3rd Edition, 2017), 203-4.

Another critic of baseball's Joseph Dorinson and Joram Warmund, Ed., Jackie Robinson: *Race, Sports and the American Dream*, M.E. Sharpe, Armonk, NY, 1999, 209.

While inspiring Black Americans, Patrick Miller & David Wiggins, Ed., *Sport & The Color Line*, Routledge, 2004, New York, 181.

It has never waned since https://today.yougov.com/topics/sport/articles-reports/2018/04/24/jackie-robinson-tops-list-sports-personalities

To say the stakes were high https://www.npr.org/templates/story/story.php?storyId=5337959

In Germany, Hitler personally http://www.ibhof.com/pages/archives/louisschmeling.html

it is believed to be the single https://www.npr.org/2006/11/25/6515548/the-fight-of-the-century-louis-vs-schmeling

More than eighty years later http://www.ibhof.com/pages/archives/louisschmeling.html

As boxing historian Thomas Hauser https://theundefeated.com/features/when-joe-louis-fought-schmeling-white-america-enthusiastically-rooted-for-a-black-man/

"Louis, who just two years earlier Patrick Miller & David Wiggins, Editors, *Sport & The Color Line*, (New York; Routledge, 2004), 138.

One of the reasons the civil rights movement Dave Zirin, *A People's History of Sports in the United States*, The New Press, New York, 2008, 139.

In a book review of a 2018 biography https://www.nytimes.com/2018/08/27/books/review/arthur-ashe-raymond-arsenault.html

As the Washington Post *reported,* https://www.washingtonpost.com/sports/tennis/us-open-winner-osaka-signs-deal-with-japanese-car-maker/2018/09/12/7a628300-b6f9-11e8-ae4f-2c1439c96d79_story.html?utm_term=.bec82f66b3e6

"[S]he is being lauded in Japan Ibid.

The New York Times *had a* https://www.nytimes.com/2018/09/09/world/asia/japan-naomi-osaka-us-open.html

Three years before Osaka https://www.japantimes.co.jp/sports/2015/10/04/general/biracial-athletes-making-strides-changing-japanese-society/#.W50qduhKiUk

The AP reporters noted that https://www.washingtonpost.com/sports/
tennis/us-open-winner-osaka-signs-deal-with-japanese-car-
maker/2018/09/12/7a628300-b6f9-11e8-ae4f-2c1439c96d79_story.
html?utm_term=.bec82f66b3e6

The University of Michigan academic Andrei S. Markovits & Lars Rensmann,
Gaming The World, Princeton University Press, Princeton & Oxford,
2010, 2.

He went so far in one study Ibid., 246.

"In formerly ethnically homogenous Ibid., 35.

...it was American sports that played Ibid., 264.

We Demand Change https://www.nytimes.com/2020/08/26/sports/
basketball/nba-boycott-bucks-magic-blake-shooting.html

Sports Fans and Women's Rights

The "Battle of the" https://en.wikipedia.org/wiki/Battle_of_the_Sexes_
(tennis)

King would become a champion Ibid.

Sports Illustrated observed that Dave Zirin, *A People's History of Sports in the
United States*, The New Press, New York, 2008, 202.

"The story of the women's movement Ibid., 21.

I have often been asked https://www.tennisforum.com/59-blast-past/204923-
billie-jean-king-remembers-life-outsider-1950s-1960s.html

Sports Fans and Religious and LGBTQ+ Tolerance

A decade before the color barrier https://www.washingtontimes.com/
news/2017/nov/29/hank-greenberg-heroic-veteran-and-baseballs-
first-/

In his memoir, Ibid.

Prominent Jewish lawyer and professor Ibid.

"Nothing illustrates the silent Andrei S. Markovits & Lars Rensmann, *Gaming
The World*, (Princeton & Oxford: Princeton University Press, 2010), 105.

"I don't think I could have come out http://time.com/5066113/gus-kenworthy-
ready-to-embrace-role-2018-winter-olympics/

"When you hear language Ibid.

"So he made a plan https://www.espn.com/olympics/story/_/id/13942305/olympic-freeskier-x-games-star-gus-kenworthy-first-openly-gay-action-sports-athlete

True to his plan, he then https://people.com/sports/winter-olympics-2018-gus-kenworthy-skiing-gay-athlete/

As he told Time http://time.com/5066113/gus-kenworthy-ready-to-embrace-role-2018-winter-olympics/

An impressed mother Ibid.

Major sponsors backed him http://time.com/5066113/gus-kenworthy-ready-to-embrace-role-2018-winter-olympics/

"That just makes me feel https://people.com/sports/winter-olympics-2018-gus-kenworthy-skiing-gay-athlete/

as he related in an op-ed for ESPN https://www.espn.com/olympics/story/_/id/27104289/how-olympian-gus-kenworthy-landed-first-hollywood-role-american-horror-story-1984

Orlando Cruz had a similarly positive https://www.newyorker.com/sports/sporting-scene/orlando-cruz-fights-to-become-boxings-first-openly-gay-champion

The notable exceptions https://www.foxsports.com/other/gallery/jason-collins-megan-rapinoe-john-amaechi-martina-navratilova-billy-bean-billie-jean-king-athetes-who-have-come-out-042913

"[A] lot of questions they ask https://www.kut.org/post/how-sports-played-role-civil-rights-movement

When All-American https://en.wikipedia.org/wiki/Michael_Sam

Sam never had that opportunity Ibid.

In 2013 NBA veteran https://www.npr.org/sections/thetwo-way/2013/04/29/179829936/nbas-jason-collins-is-first-active-player-to-come-out-as-gay

More recently, in fall 2018 https://golf.swingbyswing.com/tour/tadd-fujikawa-becomes-first-male-professional-golfer-to-come-out-as-gay/?e=487036fb16c2d15a5c957dc28a2d8c0c&e1=c3c50d132e12155e4b29ccf9e4f8021c5cdc9359&e2=b601d7c1381d38693c0b0f0df3a105f05c999a1f296e37d1863e85d483048ba0

Afterward, Fujikawa https://www.golfchannel.com/video/lynch-morning-drive-react-fujikawa-coming-out/

Sports Fans Have To Do Better

"The even greater significance those https://www.theguardian.com/sport/2018/aug/28/notes-from-an-ungrateful-athlete-why-race-and-sports-matter-in-america

Take the case of https://www.cnn.com/2013/06/05/us/trayvon-martin-shooting-fast-facts/index.html

Superstars LeBron James, Chris Bosh Cindy Boren, *Washington Post*, "When Trump attacked LeBron it had an unintended affect; other athletes speaking out," August 5, 2018

Another widely covered incident Charles Pierce, *Sports Illustrated*, October 2, 2017 p.32

I am deeply disappointed https://www.nytimes.com/2017/09/24/sports/nfl-trump-anthem-protests.html

In September 2016, two weeks https://www.cbssports.com/nfl/news/poll-majority-of-americans-disagree-with-colin-kaepernicks-protest/

Less than two years later, https://nypost.com/2018/06/07/most-voters-are-fine-with-nfl-players-anthem-kneeling-poll/

Miami Dolphins star receiver https://www.washingtonpost.com/news/early-lead/wp/2018/09/10/dolphins-kenny-stills-kneels-during-anthem-then-leads-miami-to-week-1-win/?utm_term=.07ec0ba3f7df

As a team we have decided https://www.nytimes.com/2017/09/24/sports/nfl-trump-anthem-protests.html

Likewise, NFL ratings https://www.usatoday.com/story/experience/south/my-south-experience/sports/2018/09/10/nfl-ratings-cbs-fox-improve-over-week-1-2017-nbc-dip-slightly/1255408002/

This trend continued into 2019 https://www.hollywoodreporter.com/news/whats-behind-nfls-tv-ratings-comeback-1247913

Trump again took to Twitter http://time.com/5390884/nike-sales-go-up-kaepernick-ad/

If voting with their wallets https://nypost.com/2018/09/19/nike-selling-out-of-merchandise-since-colin-kaepernick-ad/

CNBC reported that the campaign https://www.cnbc.com/2018/09/14/nikes-kaepernick-ad-should-fuel-sales-as-retailer-knows-its-consumer.html *while analysts at* https://www.cnbc.com/2018/09/18/look-for-a-kaepernick-sales-bump-in-nikes-earnings-next-week.html

Kaepernick's return could be a https://www.forbes.com/sites/kurtbadenhausen/2017/12/13/the-25-highest-paid-athletes-of-all-time/#529441944b64

New Yorker *staff writer Jelani Cobb* https://www.newyorker.com/news/daily-comment/behind-nikes-decision-to-stand-by-colin-kaepernick

Shortly after the 2018 NFL season https://www.washingtonpost.com/sports/2018/09/20/harvard-awards-colin-kaepernick-top-honor-african-african-american-studies/?utm_term=.ce7f5f5f2f9a

"Even if you've never watched https://www.vox.com/2018/4/3/17188444/lebron-james-donald-trump-michael-jordan-explained

When conservative FOX News host https://www.newsweek.com/fox-news-laura-ingraham-white-supremacist-joaquin-castro-says-amid-twitter-feud-over-migrant-1447477

Sports Fans and World Peace

"It has the power to inspire. http://db.nelsonmandela.org/speeches/pub_view.asp?pg=item&ItemID=NMS1148

British journalist John Carlin John Carlin, *Playing the Enemy*, (New York: Penguin Press, 2008), 3

When apartheid ended https://www.pri.org/stories/2014-04-27/20-years-apartheid-whats-changed-south-africa-and-what-hasnt

now it's more than 85 percent https://data.worldbank.org/indicator/EG.ELC.ACCS.ZS

The murder rate, once https://www.pri.org/stories/2014-04-27/20-years-apartheid-whats-changed-south-africa-and-what-hasnt

Black South Africans account http://www.polity.org.za/article/have-black-peoples-lives-improved-after-apartheid-2017-06-20

"If there is one thing South Africans https://www.theguardian.com/world/2014/may/06/south-africa-elections-20-years-democracy-apartheid

(Interestingly, in South Africa https://globalsportmatters.com/culture/2018/07/03/sing-stand-hand-on-heart-not-all-national-anthems-play-out-the-same/

Carlin cites numerous news reports John Carlin, Playing the Enemy, Penguin Press, New York, 2008, 245.

Archbishop Tutu, himself a Nobel Peace Prize Ibid., 245-6.

When he told his personal story https://www.theguardian.com/world/2013/dec/08/nelson-mandela-francois-pienaar-rugby-world-cup

When I watch a match in the TV https://www.nbcnews.com/news/world/iraq-s-national-soccer-team-aims-prove-nothing-can-divide-n766561

Inspired by Iran's Franklin Foer, *How Soccer Explains The World*, Harper Perennial, 2004, New York, 221.

In his bestselling 2004 globalization Ibid., 204.

"This is a common enough phenomenon Ibid., 204-5.

The team's Brazilian coach Ibid., 220-221.

Noting the growing impact https://www.nytimes.com/2002/05/26/magazine/the-world-s-game-is-not-just-a-game.html

In 2007 neighboring Iraq https://www.cnn.com/2017/07/28/football/iraq-asia-cup-2007-anniversary/index.html

In 2017 international soccer https://www.nbcnews.com/news/world/iraq-s-national-soccer-team-aims-prove-nothing-can-divide-n766561

In 2016 James M. Dorsey https://www.washingtoninstitute.org/policy-analysis/view/soccers-impact-on-middle-east-politics

In an academic article entitled Dag Tuastad, "From football riot to revolution. The political role of football in the Arab world," *Soccer & Society*, 201415:3, 376-388, DOI: 10.1080/14660970.2012.753541

English journalist and author James Montague, *When Friday Comes: Football, War, and Revolution in the Middle East*, (London: deCoubertin Books, 2013), introduction.

Egypt was the most visible Hosni Mubarak https://www.telegraph.co.uk/news/worldnews/africaandindianocean/egypt/9343310/Hosni-Mubarak-a-dictator-who-ruled-Egypt-for-three-decades.html

"[I]n Egypt people fought back James Montague, *When Friday Comes: Football, War, and Revolution in the Middle East*, (London: deCoubertin Books, 2013), introduction.

Sports, Fans, and Diplomacy

Prior to the 2018 Winter Olympic https://www.cnn.com/2018/03/09/politics/north-korea-trump-obama-bush-clinton/index.html

"Many considered it an impossible dream https://www.nytimes.com/2018/02/09/world/asia/olympics-opening-ceremony-north-korea.html

The mood of the 2018 Winter Olympic https://www.washingtonpost.com/world/as-winter-games-close-olympics-chief-lauds-diplomatic-thaw-between-the-koreas/2018/02/25/9eedf22a-18d1-11e8-930c-45838ad0d77a_story.html?noredirect=on&utm_term=.6a7d7046f464

As the New York Times *reported,* https://www.nytimes.com/2018/02/09/world/asia/olympics-opening-ceremony-north-korea.html

"In a nation like China Andrei S. Markovits & Lars Rensmann, *Gaming The World*, (Princeton & Oxford: Princeton University Press, 2010), 105.

A somewhat recent collision of sports with international affairs https://www.sbnation.com/nba/2019/10/8/20904450/nba-china-fallout-lakers-vs-nets-broadcast-streaming-tencent

The tweet, which came https://www.sportingnews.com/us/nba/news/daryl-morey-tweet-controversy-nba-china-explained/togzszxh37fi1mpw177p9bqwi

The Sports Fan and Family Ties

Professor Alan Pringle, PhD http://www.huffingtonpost.com/2015/01/30/sports-fan-mental-health-benefits_n_6565314.html

"My grandmother has a Liverpool https://www.nytimes.com/2018/08/15/opinion/revelation-of-a-liverpool-soccer-fan.html?nytapp=true

"My earliest recollections https://www.dailyrepublic.com/all-dr-news/opinion/local-opinion-columnists/sports-offer-family-bonding-experiences/

Pulitzer Prize–winning novelist Jennifer Egan http://freakonomics.com/podcast/sports-ep-1/ "How Sports Became US" (Ep. 349) 9/12/18

Journalist Shankar Vedantam https://www.npr.org/2013/10/01/228026292/examining-the-psychology-of-sports-fans

Sports and Our Brains, Part 3

In a 2018 essay entitled https://www.theatlantic.com/magazine/archive/
2018/04/be-a-fan/554081/#14

"I want the Cowboys to be Justine Gubar, *Fanaticus*, Rowman & Littlefield,
Lanham, MD, 2015, 110.

In a paper for the Journal of Wann, D. L. (2006). "Examining the potential
causal relationship between sport team identification and psychological
well-being." *Journal of Sport Behavior, 29*, 79-95.

In trying to explain https://www.psychologytoday.com/us/blog/fulfillment-
any-age/201805/the-two-emotions-drive-sports-fans

Tufts University psychologist L. Jon Wertehim & Sam Sommers, *This Is Your
Brain On Sports*, Three Rivers Press, New York, 2016, 150–159.

Sports Fans and Violence

Here is some typical hyperbole https://www.baltimoresun.com/sports/bs-md-
nfl-fan-brawls-20161005-story.html

For comparison, according https://data.cityofnewyork.us/Public-Safety/
NYPD-Arrests-Data-Historic-/8h9b-rp9u

That is one arrest per year https://nycfuture.org/research/destination-new-york

New York happens to be one of the one https://www.usatoday.com/picture-
gallery/travel/experience/america/2018/10/17/25-most-dangerous-
cities-america/1669467002/

It gets plenty of publicity, Eric Simons, *The Secret Life of Sports Fans: The Science
Of Sports Obsession*, Overlook Press, NY, 2013, 3

Dr. Aaron Smith and Hans Aaron C.T. Smith and Hans M. Westerbeek,
Sport as a Vehicle for Deploying Corporate Social Responsibility http://
citeseerx.ist.psu.edu/viewdoc/download?doi=10.1.1.472.4859&rep=
rep1&type=pdf

It's Just a Fantasy

the sports website BleacherReport https://bleacherreport.com/articles/
2036086-10-biggest-red-sox-traitors-in-franchise-history#slide10

I fell in love with football Nick Hornby, *Fever Pitch*, Penguin Group, New York,
1992, 7.

In 1961 the Oakland Raiders Gary Belsky & Neil Fine, *On The Origins of Sports: The Early History and Original Rules of Everybody's Favorite Games,* (New York: Artisan., 2016), 53.

According to Gary Belsky Ibid.

Football was not the first fantasy sport effort Ibid., 60.

($7.2 billion in 2017 https://www.usatoday.com/story/sports/fantasy/2018/08/30/fantasy-football-how-game-played-prisons-across-u-s/1109047002/

ESPN put the first https://fsta.org/research/industry-demographics/

and the next big innovation https://minnesota.cbslocal.com/2018/09/20/good-question-who-plays-fantasy-sports/

By 2017, more than 59 million https://thefsga.org/

Not surprisingly, given that https://www.nielsen.com/us/en/insights/article/2018/fantasy-is-reality-a-look-at-growing-engagement-in-fantasy-sports/

In fact, researchers found that Nicholas David Bowden, John Spinda & Jimmy Sanderson, editors, *Fantasy Sports and the Changing Sports Media Industry,* (Lanham, MD: Lexington Press, 2016), 27.

While sports fans like sports, Weiner, J., & Dwyer, B. "A new player in the game: Examining differences in motives and consumption between traditional, hybrid, and daily fantasy sport users," *Sport Marketing Quarterly,* 26(3), 2017, 142-3.

Temple University professor Joris Drayer Nicholas David Bowden, John Spinda & Jimmy Sanderson, editors, *Fantasy Sports and the Changing Sports Media Industry,* (Lanham, MD: Lexington Press, 2016), 180-81.

When Gerald Drummond is serving https://www.usatoday.com/story/sports/fantasy/2018/08/30/fantasy-football-how-game-played-prisons-across-u-s/1109047002/

The reporters' jailhouse investigation Ibid.

Former San Quentin State Prison Ibid.

In 2012, a trio of researchers Nicholas David Bowden, John Spinda & Jimmy Sanderson, editors, *Fantasy Sports and the Changing Sports Media Industry,* (Lanham, MD: Lexington Press, 2016), 75.

Clemson professor John Spinda Ibid.

University of Houston professor Andrew Baerg Ibid., 114.

The Universal Language

After many years during which http://camus-society.com/2017/11/29/albert-camus-and-football/

The Huffington Post *ran a* https://www.huffpost.com/entry/dodgers-watch-sites_b_1619068

"During the past two decades my wife Richard O. Davies, *Sports In American Life (A History)*, (Malden, MA: John Wiley and Sons, 3rd Edition, 2017), 459-60.

History professors Randy Roberts Randy Roberts & James Olson, *Winning is the Only Thing: Sports in America Since 1945*, Johns Hopkins University Press, Baltimore, 1989, 114.

"When you think of sports fans, Eric Simons, *The Secret Life of Sports Fans: The Science Of Sports Obsession*, (New York: Overlook Press, 2013), 220.

"Sport can promote Justine Gubar, *Fanaticus: Mischief and Madness in the Modern Sports Fan*, (Lanham, MD: Rowman & Littlefield, 2016), xvi.

Overtime

"Man's Joke on God" Gary Smith, *Sports Illustrated*, April 7, 2006, 54-62.

[A]t the end of the day George Will, *The Games Do Count: America's Best and Brightest on the Power of Sports*

"At the end of the day Brian Kilmeade (editor), *The Games Do Count, America's Best and Brightest on the Power of Sports*, (New York: Regan Books, 2004), 61.

AVON PUBLIC LIBRARY
PO BOX 977 / 200 BENCHMARK RD
AVON CO 81620 (970)949-6797